A Textbook of Receptor Pharmacology

A Textbook of Receptor Pharmacology

By

Souravh Bais and Renu Kumari

Cambridge
Scholars
Publishing

A Textbook of Receptor Pharmacology

By Souravh Bais and Renu Kumari

This book first published 2026

Cambridge Scholars Publishing

Lady Stephenson Library, Newcastle upon Tyne, NE6 2PA, UK

British Library Cataloguing in Publication Data
A catalogue record for this book is available from the British Library

ISBN: 978-1-0364-7467-6
ISBN (Ebook): 978-1-0364-7468-3

TABLE OF CONTENTS

PREFACE

Receptor pharmacology represents the unifying framework through which the actions of drugs, hormones, neurotransmitters, and endogenous mediators can be understood at the molecular, cellular, and systemic levels. With the rapid expansion of receptor biology—from classical receptor theory to contemporary concepts such as biased agonism, receptor crosstalk, and translational signaling—there is a growing need for a structured, receptor-centric textbook that integrates fundamental principles with clinically relevant receptor systems. *A Text Book of Receptor Pharmacology* has been conceived to address this need.

The present book is systematically organized to provide both conceptual clarity and practical relevance. It begins with the *Principles of Receptor Pharmacology*, establishing a strong foundation in receptor–ligand interactions, affinity, efficacy, signal transduction, dose–response relationships, receptor regulation, and clinical pharmacodynamics. This foundational framework is essential for understanding the diverse receptor families discussed in subsequent chapters.

Following the introductory principles, the book adopts a receptor-wise approach, with dedicated chapters on major G-protein-coupled receptors, ligand-gated ion channels, enzyme-linked receptors, nuclear receptors, and emerging receptor classes. Each receptor chapter—covering systems such as adenosine, adrenergic, angiotensin, apelin, bile acid, bombesin, bradykinin, calcitonin, calcium-sensing, cannabinoid, chemerin, chemokine, and several other clinically significant receptors—is structured to include definition, classification, signaling mechanisms, pharmacological actions, therapeutic indications, contraindications, and clinical relevance. Wherever appropriate, recent experimental insights and clinically meaningful examples have been incorporated to strengthen translational understanding.

Special emphasis has been placed on linking receptor mechanisms to disease pathophysiology and pharmacotherapy. Concepts such as receptor subtype selectivity, functional selectivity, receptor desensitization, and regulation have been contextualized with real-world clinical scenarios, making the content particularly useful for pharmacy, medical, and life-science students, as well as for researchers engaged in drug discovery and experimental pharmacology.

The content and presentation of this textbook reflect the authors' combined academic experience in pharmacology teaching, experimental research, and interdisciplinary collaboration across neuropharmacology, metabolic disorders, inflammation, and phytopharmacology. The intent has been to maintain scientific rigor while ensuring readability and pedagogical coherence.

This book is primarily intended for undergraduate and postgraduate students of Pharmacy (B.Pharm, M.Pharm, and Pharm.D), Medicine, Nursing, Biotechnology, and Life Sciences. It will also serve as a valuable reference for academicians, researchers, and clinicians seeking a concise yet comprehensive resource on receptor-based pharmacology.

We sincerely hope that *A Text Book of Receptor Pharmacology* will contribute meaningfully to pharmacological education, foster conceptual depth, and inspire readers to appreciate the central role of receptors in modern therapeutics and drug development.

— The Authors
Dr Souravh Bais
Mrs Renu Kumari

BOOK BLURB

A Text Book of Receptor Pharmacology provides a comprehensive, receptor-oriented exploration of drug action at the molecular and cellular levels. Beginning with fundamental principles of receptor pharmacodynamics, the book systematically examines a wide spectrum of clinically and experimentally important receptor systems, including GPCRs, ion channels, enzyme-linked receptors, nuclear receptors, and emerging receptor targets.

Each chapter integrates receptor classification, signaling mechanisms, pharmacological actions, therapeutic indications, contraindications, and clinical relevance, offering a balanced blend of theory and application. With dedicated coverage of receptors such as adenosine, adrenergic, angiotensin, apelin, bile acid, cannabinoid, chemokine, calcium-sensing, and several neuro- and immunopharmacological receptors, this textbook reflects the contemporary scope of receptor science.

Written by experienced pharmacology academicians and researchers, the book is designed to support undergraduate and postgraduate education while also serving as a practical reference for researchers and professionals. Its structured presentation and emphasis on translational relevance make it an essential resource for understanding receptor-based therapeutics in modern pharmacology.

AUTHOR BIOGRAPHIES

Dr. Souravh Bais

Dr. Souravh Bais is a Professor of Pharmacology with more than 14 years of teaching, research, and academic leadership experience. He holds a PhD in Pharmacology, an M.Pharm in Pharmacology, and an MA in Clinical Psychology, reflecting his strong interdisciplinary orientation. He is currently associated with SAGE University, Indore, where he is actively involved in undergraduate, postgraduate, and doctoral teaching and research supervision.

Dr. Bais has made significant contributions to neuropharmacology, metabolic disorders, obesity, inflammation, ethnopharmacology, and experimental therapeutics. He has authored over 65 research and review articles in reputed national and international journals and has contributed book chapters, patents, and copyrights in areas spanning drug discovery, pharmacological innovation, and AI-assisted biomedical applications.

He serves as a reviewer and editor for several international journals and is a member of professional bodies including the British Pharmacological Society, ASPET, and APTI. His academic interests strongly emphasize receptor pharmacology, signal transduction mechanisms, and the translation of receptor-based concepts into rational pharmacotherapy and drug development.

Mrs. Renu Kumari

Mrs. Renu Kumari is an Assistant Professor of Pharmacology associated with the Institute of Pharmaceutical Sciences, SAGE University, Indore, and Government Asthang Ayurvedic College, Indore, Madhya Pradesh, India. She is currently pursuing her PhD in Pharmacology and is actively engaged in teaching and experimental research.

Her research expertise includes neuropharmacology, metabolic and neurometabolic disorders, phytopharmacology, behavioral neuroscience, and inflammatory mechanisms. She has authored more than 15 publications in peer-reviewed international journals and has contributed book chapters, patents, and copyrights. Her experimental work extensively utilizes in-vivo animal models to investigate neurodegeneration, obesity, seizure disorders, and receptor-mediated pharmacological interventions, with a particular focus on plant-derived bioactive compounds.

Mrs. Kumari's scholarly work has received notable citations, reflecting her growing impact in pharmacological research. Through her academic and research activities, she continues to contribute to receptor-based understanding of disease mechanisms and therapeutic strategies, particularly at the interface of natural products and modern pharmacology.

LIST OF FIGURES

LIST OF TABLES

LIST OF ABBREVIATIONS

ACE	Angiotensin Converting Enzyme
AD	Alzheimer's Disease
ADRs	Adverse Drug Reactions
ARB	Angiotensin Receptor Blocker
AT_1R	Angiotensin II Type 1 Receptor
AT_2R	Angiotensin II Type 2 Receptor
ATP	Adenosine Triphosphate
BBB	Blood–Brain Barrier
BK	Bradykinin
BP	Blood Pressure
CaSR	Calcium-Sensing Receptor
cAMP	Cyclic Adenosine Monophosphate
CB1	Cannabinoid Receptor Type 1
CB2	Cannabinoid Receptor Type 2
CCB	Calcium Channel Blocker
CCR	CC Chemokine Receptor
CGRP	Calcitonin Gene-Related Peptide
CKD	Chronic Kidney Disease
CNS	Central Nervous System
COPD	Chronic Obstructive Pulmonary Disease
CXCR	CXC Chemokine Receptor
EC_{50}	Effective Concentration 50%
ED_{50}	Effective Dose 50%
EGFR	Epidermal Growth Factor Receptor
FXR	Farnesoid X Receptor
Gi/Gs/Gq	G-Protein Subtypes
GLP-1	Glucagon-Like Peptide-1
GPCR	G-Protein-Coupled Receptor
GRP	Gastrin-Releasing Peptide
HIV	Human Immunodeficiency Virus
IBD	Inflammatory Bowel Disease
IL	Interleukin
IP_3	Inositol Triphosphate
KD	Dissociation Constant
MAPK	Mitogen-Activated Protein Kinase
MS	Multiple Sclerosis

NAFLD	Non-Alcoholic Fatty Liver Disease
NASH	Non-Alcoholic Steatohepatitis
NMDA	N-Methyl-D-Aspartate
NO	Nitric Oxide
PTH	Parathyroid Hormone
RAAS	Renin–Angiotensin–Aldosterone System
ROS	Reactive Oxygen Species
SVT	Supraventricular Tachycardia
TD_{50}	Toxic Dose 50%
TGR5	G-Protein-Coupled Bile Acid Receptor 1
THC	Tetrahydrocannabinol
TNF-α	Tumor Necrosis Factor Alpha

CHAPTER 1

PRINCIPLES OF RECEPTOR PHARMACOLOGY

Introduction: The Foundation of Pharmacodynamics

Receptor pharmacology is the bedrock of modern medicine, a discipline that seeks to understand how chemical substances, both endogenous and synthetic, interact with biological systems to produce a physiological effect. At its core, this field is built upon the concept of the receptor, a macromolecule—typically a protein—that serves as a cellular target for signaling molecules. These receptors are the molecular sentinels of the cell, poised to receive specific signals and translate them into a cascade of intracellular events that ultimately alter cellular function. The essence of pharmacology lies in the deliberate manipulation of these interactions to treat disease, a principle summarized by the key-and-lock model, which posits that a drug must have a specific structural complementarity with its receptor to elicit a response.

This chapter delves into the intricate world of receptor pharmacology, exploring the nature of receptor-ligand interactions, the diverse mechanisms of signal transduction, the classification of drugs based on their receptor effects, and the quantitative methods used to measure and predict drug action. By understanding these principles, we can appreciate the precision with which modern drugs are designed and administered, paving the way for more targeted and effective therapeutic interventions.

Receptor-Ligand Interactions: Affinity and Specificity

The initial step in a pharmacological response is the binding of a ligand—any molecule that binds to a receptor—to its receptor. This interaction is governed by several fundamental principles.

Affinity

Affinity is a measure of the strength of the binding between a ligand and its receptor. A high-affinity ligand binds strongly and readily to its receptor, even at low concentrations, while a low-affinity ligand requires a higher concentration to achieve the same level of binding. This relationship is often quantified by the dissociation constant, KD, which represents the concentration of a ligand required to occupy 50% of the available receptors at equilibrium. A lower KD value indicates a higher affinity.

The binding of a ligand to a receptor is a reversible process governed by the law of mass action. The equilibrium between the ligand (L), the receptor (R), and the ligand-receptor complex (LR) is described by the equation:

$L+R \rightleftharpoons LR$

The KD is a ratio of the off-rate constant (koff) to the on-rate constant (kon), where koff is the rate at which the complex dissociates and kon is the rate at which it forms.

KD=[LR][L][R]=konkoff

Selectivity and Specificity

Receptor selectivity refers to the ability of a drug to bind to a specific type of receptor. A highly selective drug binds only to its intended target, minimizing off-target effects and reducing the risk of side effects. Specificity, while often used interchangeably with selectivity, can also refer to the ability of a receptor to discriminate between different ligands. This is a crucial concept in drug design, as subtle changes in a drug's chemical structure can dramatically alter its selectivity, leading to a different therapeutic profile.

Signal Transduction Mechanisms: From Binding to Response

Once a ligand binds to its receptor, the signal must be transduced from the cell's exterior to its interior. Receptors are classified into four main families based on their structure and signal transduction mechanism.

1. Ligand-Gated Ion Channels (Ionotropic Receptors)

These receptors are also ion channels. Upon ligand binding, a conformational change occurs, opening or closing the channel and allowing specific ions (e.g., Na+,K+,Ca2+,Cl−) to flow across the cell membrane. This rapid change in ion concentration alters the cell's membrane potential, leading to a rapid response, such as a nerve impulse.

The nicotinic acetylcholine receptor is a classic example of this type, mediating fast synaptic transmission at the neuromuscular junction.

2. G-Protein Coupled Receptors (GPCRs)

GPCRs constitute the largest and most diverse family of receptors, responsible for mediating the effects of a vast array of signaling molecules, including hormones, neurotransmitters, and light. These receptors have a characteristic structure with seven transmembrane helices. When a ligand binds to a GPCR, it induces a conformational change that activates an intracellular G-protein (guanosine nucleotide-binding protein). The G-protein, in turn, can activate or inhibit various intracellular enzymes or ion channels, leading to the generation of second messengers such as cyclic AMP (cAMP) or inositol trisphosphate (IP3). This signal amplification cascade allows a single ligand-binding event to produce a large and sustained cellular response.

3. Enzyme-Linked Receptors

These receptors are transmembrane proteins with an extracellular ligand-binding domain and an intracellular enzyme domain. Ligand binding often causes the receptor to dimerize, activating the intrinsic enzyme activity of the intracellular domain. The most common form is the receptor tyrosine kinase, which phosphorylates tyrosine residues on target proteins. This phosphorylation cascade initiates a series of downstream signaling events that regulate cell growth, differentiation, and metabolism. The insulin receptor is a well-known example.

4. Intracellular Receptors

Unlike the other three families, intracellular receptors are located within the cytoplasm or nucleus of the cell. Their ligands are typically small, lipid-soluble molecules, such as steroid hormones and thyroid hormones, which can diffuse across the cell membrane. Once inside, the ligand binds to its receptor, and the complex then translocates to the nucleus, where it acts as a transcription factor, directly modulating gene expression. This mechanism is slower than the others, taking hours to days to manifest a full effect, but its effects are often long-lasting.

Drug-Receptor Relationships: Agonists and Antagonists

The classification of drugs is not only based on their chemical structure but also on their effect on receptor function.

Agonists

An agonist is a drug that binds to a receptor and activates it, producing a pharmacological response. Agonists have both affinity for the receptor and intrinsic efficacy, which is a measure of the drug's ability to produce a maximum response upon binding.

- ❖ **Full Agonists:** These drugs produce the maximum possible biological response when they occupy all or a fraction of the available receptors. Their intrinsic efficacy is considered to be 1.
- ❖ **Partial Agonists:** These drugs can bind to and activate a receptor but are unable to elicit the maximum possible response, even at high concentrations. They have an intrinsic efficacy between 0 and 1.
- ❖ **Inverse Agonists:** Some receptors exhibit a basal level of constitutive activity in the absence of a ligand. An inverse agonist binds to this receptor and stabilizes it in an inactive conformation, thereby reducing the basal activity.

Antagonists

An antagonist is a drug that binds to a receptor but does not activate it. Its primary effect is to block the binding of an agonist and thus prevent a response. Antagonists have affinity but no intrinsic efficacy (efficacy = 0).

- **Competitive Antagonists:** These antagonists bind reversibly to the same site as the agonist. The effect can be overcome by increasing the concentration of the agonist. On a dose-response curve, this shifts the curve to the right without affecting the maximum response (Emax).
- **Non-Competitive Antagonists:** These antagonists bind to a different site on the receptor (an allosteric site) or to the agonist-binding site irreversibly. This reduces the number of functional receptors available for the agonist, thereby decreasing the maximum response (Emax) of the agonist without affecting its potency.

Allosteric Modulators

Allosteric modulators bind to a site on the receptor that is distinct from the agonist-binding site. They do not have an effect on their own but can alter the receptor's response to an agonist. Positive allosteric modulators enhance the agonist's effect, while negative allosteric modulators diminish it.

Quantifying Drug-Receptor Interactions: Dose-Response Curves

The relationship between the dose of a drug and the magnitude of the pharmacological response is typically represented by a dose-response curve.

Potency vs. Efficacy

- **Potency:** This refers to the amount of drug required to produce a given effect. It is often expressed as the EC50 (effective concentration 50), which is the concentration of a drug that produces 50% of the maximum possible response. A drug with a lower EC50 is more potent.
- **Efficacy:** This refers to the maximum response a drug can produce, regardless of the dose. It is a measure of the drug's intrinsic activity. A drug with higher efficacy is more effective at producing a strong response.

Therapeutic Index

The therapeutic index is a ratio that compares the dose of a drug that produces a therapeutic effect to the dose that causes a toxic effect. It is a measure of a drug's safety.

TherapeuticIndex=ED50/TD50

where TD50 is the toxic dose for 50% of the population and ED50 is the effective dose for 50% of the population. A higher therapeutic index indicates a safer drug.

Receptor Regulation and Clinical Relevance

Receptors are not static entities; their number and sensitivity can be regulated by chronic exposure to drugs or endogenous ligands.

- **Desensitization:** A rapid decrease in a receptor's response to a ligand, often due to phosphorylation of the receptor, which uncouples it from its signaling pathway.
- **Down-regulation:** A more gradual decrease in the number of receptors on the cell surface, often in response to chronic exposure to high concentrations of an agonist.
- **Up-regulation:** An increase in the number of receptors on the cell surface, often in response to chronic exposure to an antagonist or a lack of the endogenous ligand.

These regulatory mechanisms have significant clinical implications, influencing the development of tolerance to a drug or the withdrawal symptoms that occur when a drug is stopped abruptly. For instance, chronic use of opioid agonists can lead to receptor down-regulation, requiring higher doses to achieve the same effect.

Summary

Receptor pharmacology provides the fundamental framework for understanding drug action. By elucidating the intricate interactions between ligands and their protein targets, we can design drugs with enhanced affinity, selectivity, and efficacy. The study of dose-response relationships, receptor regulation, and signal transduction cascades allows us to predict a drug's therapeutic and toxic effects, paving the way for the development of safer and more effective medicines. The principles outlined in this chapter are not merely theoretical constructs; they are the guiding force behind every new drug discovery, offering a precise and powerful means to manipulate biological systems for the betterment of human health. As we continue to uncover the complexities of cellular signaling, receptor pharmacology will remain at the forefront of pharmaceutical innovation, driving progress toward personalized and highly targeted therapies.

CHAPTER 2

ADENOSINE RECEPTORS

Adenosine receptors are a group of G-protein-coupled receptors (GPCRs) that mediate the physiological effects of adenosine, a purine nucleoside involved in various cellular processes. They are widely expressed in mammalian tissues and regulate numerous biological functions, including cardiovascular, neurological, renal, and immune responses.

Classification of Adenosine Receptors

Adenosine receptors are classified into four subtypes:

1. **A1**: Found in the heart, brain, and adipose tissue.
2. **A2A**: Predominantly in the brain (especially the basal ganglia), vasculature, and immune cells.
3. **A2B**: Expressed in the vasculature, gastrointestinal tract, lungs, and immune cells.
4. **A3**: Present in the brain, heart, liver, and immune cells.

Each subtype has distinct tissue distribution, pharmacological properties, and physiological roles.

Pharmacological Actions

1. **A1 Receptors**: it Inhibit adenylyl cyclase via Gi proteins, decreasing cyclic AMP (cAMP) levels.
   Effects: Negative chronotropic and dromotropic actions in the heart, inhibition of neurotransmitter release, and renal vasoconstriction.
2. **A2A Receptors**: it Stimulate adenylyl cyclase via Gs proteins, increasing cAMP levels.
   Effects: Vasodilation, inhibition of platelet aggregation, and modulation of dopamine signaling.

3. **A2B Receptors**: Similar to A2A receptors but require higher adenosine concentrations for activation.
   Effects: Bronchodilation, vascular relaxation, and pro-inflammatory or anti-inflammatory responses depending on the context.
4. **A3 Receptors**: it coupled with Gi and Gq proteins, affecting intracellular calcium levels and cAMP.
   Effects: Cardioprotection, anti-inflammatory responses, and regulation of mast cell degranulation.

Indications

1. **A1 Receptor Agonists**: these are used for supraventricular tachycardia (SVT) management (e.g., adenosine itself) and play potential role in neuroprotection and analgesia.
2. **A2A Receptor Agonists**: these drugs are used for management of Parkinson's disease (inhibition of overactive dopaminergic pathways) and anti-inflammatory and vasodilatory effects.
3. **A2B Receptor Antagonists**: its role is under investigation for asthma and chronic obstructive pulmonary disease (COPD).
4. **A3 Receptor Agonists**: Experimental use in cancer therapy and inflammatory diseases like rheumatoid arthritis.

Contraindications

1. **A1 Receptor Agonists**: Contraindicated in patients with second- or third-degree AV block without a pacemaker. Use cautiously in asthma due to potential bronchoconstriction.
2. **A2A Receptor Agonists**: Contraindicated in hypotension or bleeding disorders due to vasodilatory effects.
3. **A2B Receptor Antagonists**: No absolute contraindications yet established, as these are primarily experimental.
4. **A3 Receptor Agonists**: Avoid in conditions where excessive immune modulation could worsen the disease.

Clinical Importance

Receptor structure/function in drug design (adenosine A_2A receptor)

Summary:A case study showing how stabilised GPCR structure (adenosine A_2A receptor) enabled drug design, linking receptor structure, ligand binding, pharmacology.

Relevance: Useful for method/educational case: "how understanding receptor structure aids pharmacotherapy". Could be used in a chapter on drug development linked to receptor pharmacology.

Citation: Andrews SP, Tehan B. Stabilised G protein-coupled receptors in structure-based drug design: a case study with adenosine A_2A receptor. Med Chem Comm. 2013;4(1):52-67. doi:10.1039/C2MD20164J. RSC Publishing.

CHAPTER 3

ADHESION CLASS OF GPCRS

The adhesion class of G-protein-coupled receptors (GPCRs) is a group of receptors that are involved in mediating cell-cell interactions, cellular adhesion, and signal transduction. These receptors are characterized by their large extracellular domains, which are involved in binding to extracellular matrix components or other cell adhesion molecules. They play crucial roles in various physiological processes, including immune responses, neuronal development, and tissue organization.

Definition of Adhesion Class GPCRs

Adhesion GPCRs are a distinct subclass of GPCRs that are characterized by a long extracellular region that includes multiple immunoglobulin-like (Ig-like) domains and/or other adhesion-like domains. These receptors are involved in mediating intercellular communication, often in the context of cell adhesion, migration, and signaling in both development and immune responses. They have a unique structural configuration and, unlike other GPCRs, their activation involves more complex mechanisms, often requiring conformational changes that are triggered by the interaction with ligands or the extracellular matrix.

Classification of Adhesion Class GPCRs

The adhesion GPCRs are typically classified into the following subgroups based on their structure and function:

1. **Family 1** (also known as **Class B** adhesion GPCRs): These are the best-known group, which includes receptors involved in various immune and developmental processes.
   Example: L1CAM (L1 Cell Adhesion Molecule), which is involved in neural development and synaptic plasticity.

2. **Family 2** (also known as **Class C** adhesion GPCRs): These receptors are involved in neuronal development and immune cell function.
   Example: GPR56 (adhesion GPCR), which plays a role in neurodevelopment and tissue organization.
3. **Family 3** (also known as **Class D** adhesion GPCRs): These include receptors that play roles in endothelial cells and immune responses.
   Example: GPR97, which is involved in the regulation of inflammatory responses.
4. **Family 4** (also known as **Class E** adhesion GPCRs): A relatively less explored subgroup with specialized roles.
   Example: GPR113, implicated in immune response and some forms of cancer.

Pharmacological Actions

The pharmacological actions of adhesion GPCRs are highly diverse and depend on the specific receptor subtype and itssignaling pathway. Here are some general pharmacological actions:

1. **Regulation of cell adhesion and migration**: Many adhesion GPCRs play key roles in cellular interactions, which are critical for immune responses, wound healing, and cancer metastasis.
   Example: GPR56 in neurons regulates adhesion and migration during brain development.
2. **Immune system modulation**: Adhesion GPCRs, such as T cell immunoglobulin and mucin domain (TIM) receptors, modulate immune cell adhesion and activation, contributing to immune tolerance or activation during infections and autoimmune diseases.
3. **Neurodevelopment and neuronal signalling**: Adhesion GPCRs, like **L1CAM**, regulate neuronal growth, axon guidance, and synaptic plasticity, which are important for proper nervous system function.
4. **Regulation of vascular development and inflammation**: Receptors such as GPR56 influence endothelial cell behavior, vascular formation, and inflammation.
5. **Tissue homeostasis**: Some adhesion GPCRs play roles in maintaining tissue integrity, such as through regulating the extracellular matrix and the epithelial-mesenchymal transition.

Indications for Adhesion GPCR Modulation

The therapeutic potential of adhesion GPCRs is under investigation for several indications, including:

1. **Cancer Therapy**: Targeting adhesion GPCRs like **GPR56** may help in modulating tumor progression, metastasis, and tumor microenvironment.
2. **Autoimmune and Inflammatory Diseases**: Modulating immune-related adhesion GPCRs may provide therapeutic benefit in autoimmune diseases (e.g., multiple sclerosis, rheumatoid arthritis).
3. **Neurodevelopmental Disorders**: Manipulating adhesion GPCRs like **L1CAM** may provide treatments for developmental disorders, such as those related to neuronal adhesion, migration, and synaptic plasticity.
4. **Wound Healing and Tissue Repair**: Adhesion GPCRs play roles in regulating wound healing by modulating cell migration and tissue remodeling.

Contraindications

Although adhesion GPCRs present potential therapeutic targets, there are also concerns and possible contraindications in targeting these receptors due to their broad roles in normal cellular function:

1. **Cancer Therapy**: Inhibiting adhesion GPCRs involved in tumor cell migration might not be suitable for all cancer types and could potentially disrupt normal tissue repair processes.
2. **Immune Suppression**: Inhibiting adhesion GPCRs involved in immune cell activation may impair the immune response, making it inappropriate for patients with compromised immune systems or chronic infections.
3. **Neurological Disorders**: Modulation of adhesion GPCRs involved in neuronal migration or axonal guidance could have unintended effects on brain development, potentially exacerbating conditions like neurodevelopmental disorders or epilepsy.
4. **Vascular Effects**: Targeting adhesion GPCRs involved in vascular development and inflammation may lead to unwanted side effects like excessive vascular leakage or inflammation, especially in diseases like atherosclerosis.

CHAPTER 4

ADRENOCEPTORS (ADRENERGIC RECEPTORS)

Adrenoceptors are G-protein-coupled receptors (GPCRs) that mediate the physiological responses to catecholamines (e.g., adrenaline and noradrenaline). These receptors play a key role in the sympathetic nervous system, regulating cardiovascular, respiratory, metabolic, and central nervous system functions.

Definition of Adrenoceptors

Adrenoceptors are membrane-bound receptors activated by adrenaline (epinephrine) and noradrenaline (norepinephrine). They transduce signals via G-proteins to elicit various physiological effects, such as vasoconstriction, bronchodilation, and metabolic regulation.

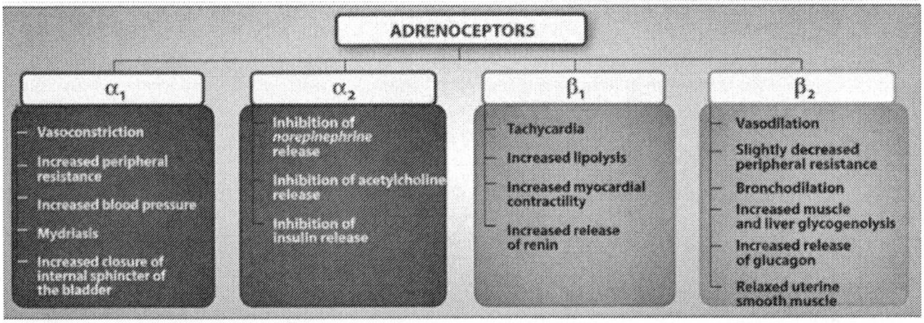

Fig 3.1 Types ans effects of Adrenoreceptors.

Classification of Adrenoceptors

Adrenoceptors are classified into two main families and further subdivided based on their pharmacological and functional characteristics:

1. **Alpha (α) Adrenoceptors**:
   - **α1**: Coupled to Gq proteins, primarily mediating smooth muscle contraction.
   - **α2**: Coupled to Gi proteins, inhibiting adenylyl cyclase and decreasing cAMP levels.
2. **Beta (β) Adrenoceptors**:
   - **β1**: Coupled to Gs proteins, stimulating adenylyl cyclase and increasing cAMP levels, primarily in the heart.
   - **β2**: Coupled to Gs proteins, causing smooth muscle relaxation, primarily in the bronchi and vasculature.
   - **β3**: Coupled to Gs proteins, primarily involved in lipolysis in adipose tissue.

Pharmacological Actions

1. **Alpha (α) Adrenoceptors**:
   - **α1**: Vasoconstriction of arterioles and veins. Contraction of smooth muscles (e.g., bladder sphincter, iris dilator muscle).
   - **α2**: Inhibition of norepinephrine release (autoreceptor function), Platelet aggregation and reduction in insulin secretion.
2. **Beta (β) Adrenoceptors**:
   - **β1**: it produces Positive inotropic (increased contractility) and chronotropic (increased heart rate) effects on the heart and causes Renin release from the kidneys.
   - **β2**: it causes
     - Bronchodilation.
     - Vasodilation of skeletal muscle vasculature.
     - Glycogenolysis and gluconeogenesis in the liver.
     - Uterine relaxation.
   - **β3**: it causes
     - Lipolysis in adipose tissue.
     - Relaxation of the bladder detrusor muscle.

Indications

1. **Alpha (α) Agonists**:
   - **α1 Agonists**: are used in hypotension, nasal congestion (e.g., phenylephrine).
   - **α2 Agonists**: are used in hypertension, sedation, and pain management (e.g., clonidine).

2. **Beta (β) Agonists**:
    - **β1 Agonists**: Used in heart failure and cardiogenic shock to improve cardiac output (e.g., dobutamine).
    - **β2 Agonists**: Used in asthma and chronic obstructive pulmonary disease (COPD) to promote bronchodilation (e.g., salbutamol, terbutaline).
    - **β3 Agonists**: Used for overactive bladder to relax the detrusor muscle (e.g., mirabegron).
3. **Alpha (α) Antagonists**:
    - **α1 Antagonists**: Used in hypertension and benign prostatic hyperplasia (e.g., prazosin, tamsulosin).
    - **α2 Antagonists**: Experimental use in depression and cognitive enhancement.
4. **Beta (β) Antagonists (Beta-Blockers)**:
    - Non-selective or selective antagonists are used in hypertension, angina, heart failure, arrhythmias, and anxiety (e.g., propranolol, metoprolol, carvedilol).

Contraindications

1. **Alpha (α) Agonists**:
    - **α1 Agonists**: these are contraindicated in severe hypertension or patients with pheochromocytoma.
    - **α2 Agonists**: these drugs avoid in severe bradycardia or patients prone to hypotension.
2. **Beta (β) Agonists**:
    - **β1 Agonists**: these drugs contraindicated in tachyarrhythmias or conditions where increased myocardial oxygen demand is harmful.
    - **β2 Agonists**: these drugs avoided in patients with severe cardiovascular disease due to risk of tachycardia.
3. **Alpha (α) Antagonists**: these drugs avoided in patients with a history of postural hypotension.
4. **Beta (β) Antagonists**: these drugs contraindicated in:
    - Severe bradycardia or heart block.
    - Asthma or severe COPD (for non-selective beta-blockers).
    - Decompensated heart failure.

Clinical Importance

Role: β-Adrenergic receptors and β-blockers

Citation: Frishman WH, Saunders E. β-Adrenergic blockers. J Clin Hypertens (Greenwich). 2011 Aug;13(9):649-653. doi:10.1111/j.1751-7176.2011.00515.x. PMC

Summary: Overview of ¬β adrenergic receptor pharmacology, the role of β-blockers in hypertension, heart failure and other indications; mechanism (antagonism at β_1/β_2) etc.

Clinical Relevance: Good for a clinical case: e.g., "60 yo female with ischemic heart disease and hypertension is started on metoprolol (β_1-selective antagonist) … discuss receptor subtype selectivity, pharmacologic consequences (bronchospasm risk if β_2 blocked)

CHAPTER 5

ANGIOTENSIN RECEPTORS

Angiotensin receptors are G-protein-coupled receptors (GPCRs) that mediate the physiological and pathological effects of angiotensin II, a key hormone in the renin-angiotensin-aldosterone system (RAAS). These receptors regulate blood pressure, fluid balance, and cardiovascular remodeling.

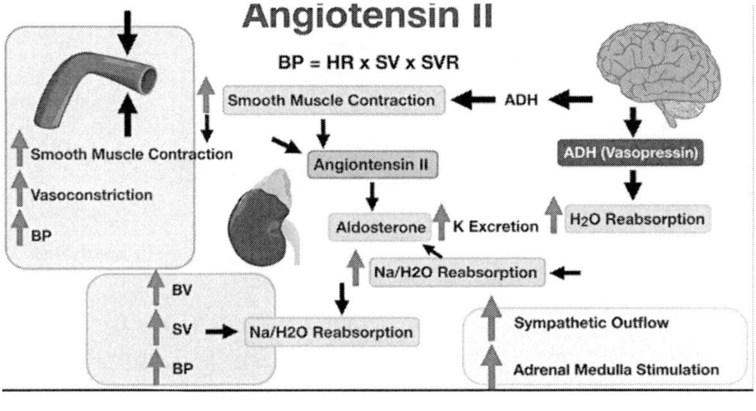

Fig 4.1 Release and mechanaism of action of Angiotenisin-II.

Definition of Angiotensin Receptors

Angiotensin receptors are cell surface receptors that primarily respond to angiotensin II, a potent vasoconstrictor. They play a central role in cardiovascular, renal, and endocrine systems by regulating vascular tone, sodium retention, and cell growth.

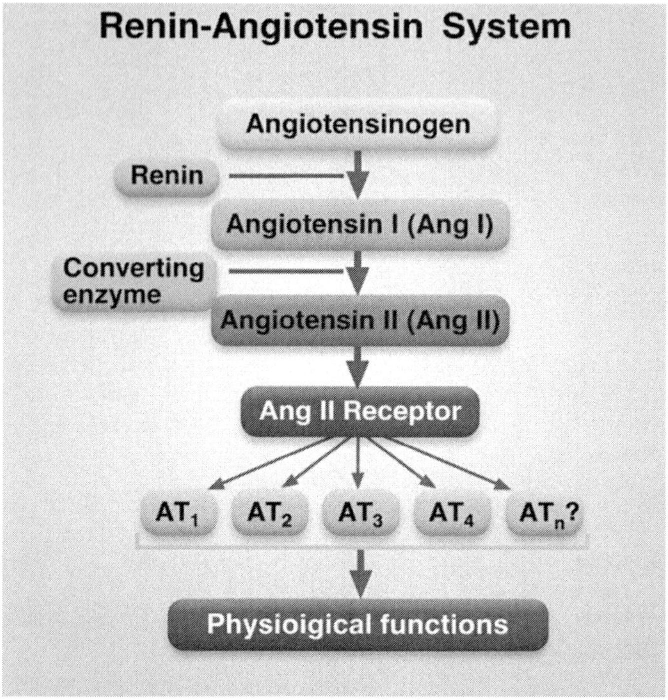

Fig. 4.2 Renin Angiotensin System

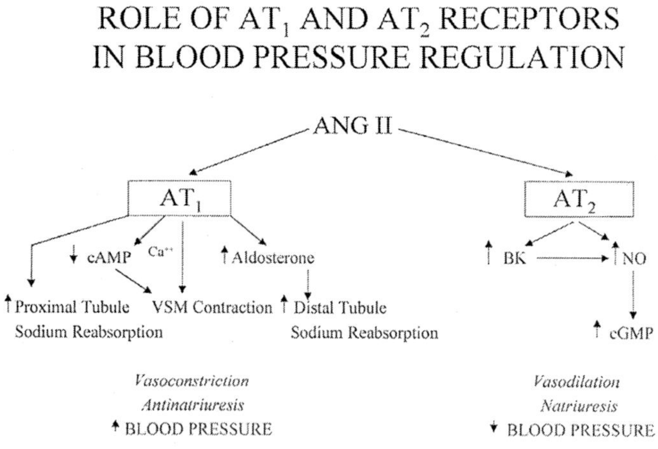

Fig. 4.3 Physiological actions of RAS activation.

Classification of Angiotensin Receptors

Angiotensin receptors are classified into two main subtypes, with distinct functions:

1. **Angiotensin II Type 1 Receptor (AT_1R)**: Predominantly mediates the classical effects of angiotensin II, such as vasoconstriction, sodium retention, and pro-inflammatory responses.
2. **Angiotensin II Type 2 Receptor (AT_2R)**: Generally, counteracts the effects of AT_1R, promoting vasodilation, anti-inflammatory effects, and tissue repair.

Pharmacological Actions

1. **AT_1R (Pro-Hypertensive Actions)**:
   - **Vasoconstriction**: Increases vascular resistance and blood pressure.
   - **Aldosterone Secretion**: Enhances sodium and water retention by the kidneys.
   - **Cellular Growth**: Promotes smooth muscle and cardiac hypertrophy.
   - **Pro-inflammatory Effects**: Stimulates production of cytokines and reactive oxygen species (ROS).
2. **AT_2R (Protective Actions)**:
   - **Vasodilation**: Reduces vascular resistance.
   - **Anti-inflammatory Effects**: Suppresses cytokine production.
   - **Anti-fibrotic and Anti-proliferative Actions**: Limits tissue fibrosis and cellular growth.
   - **Neuroprotection**: Supports nerve regeneration and repair.

Indications

1. **Angiotensin Receptor Blockers (ARBs)**:
   - Selectively block AT_1R, preventing angiotensin II-mediated harmful effects.
   - Examples: Losartan, Valsartan, Telmisartan, Candesartan.
2. **Conditions Treated with ARBs**:
   - **Hypertension**: To lower blood pressure by inhibiting vasoconstriction.
   - **Heart Failure**: To reduce afterload and prevent ventricular remodeling.

- **Chronic Kidney Disease (CKD)**: To slow progression by reducing intraglomerular pressure.
- **Post-Myocardial Infarction**: To prevent cardiac remodeling and improve outcomes.

Contraindications

1. **Absolute Contraindications**:
   - **Pregnancy**: ARBs are teratogenic and can cause fetal toxicity.
   - **Severe Bilateral Renal Artery Stenosis**: Risk of acute kidney failure.
   - **Hypersensitivity**: Known allergy to ARBs.
2. **Relative Contraindications**:
   - **Hyperkalemia**: ARBs may increase serum potassium levels.
   - **Severe Dehydration**: Risk of hypotension due to reduced circulating volume.

Clinical Importance

Role: Biased agonism / functional selectivity at the angiotensin II type 1 receptor

Summary: This research explores how cyclic analogs of ¬Angiotensin II type 1 receptor (AT_1R) ligands selectively activate certain downstream pathways (e.g., $G_{(q/11)}$ vs β-arrestin) thereby illustrating biased agonism.

Relevance: Great for a chapter on "biased signaling" or "functional selectivity in receptors" — you might present a case vignette: patient treated with AT_1R-blocking drug but differing side-effect profiles due to pathway bias.

Citation:St-Pierre D, Cabana J, Holleran BJ, Besserer-Offroy É, Escher E, Guillemette G, Lavigne P, Leduc R. Angiotensin II cyclic analogs as tools to investigate AT_1R biased signaling mechanisms. BioRxiv/Preprint 2019. doi:10.1101/582595. arXiv

Role: Clinical pharmacology of angiotensin II receptor antagonists

Summary: A review of the class of ¬Losartan (an AT_1R antagonist) and related drugs: mechanism (antagonism of angiotensin II type 1 receptor), pharmacokinetics, clinical efficacy in hypertension.

Relevance: Useful for a straightforward receptor-based therapeutic case study: e.g., a patient with hypertension treated with losartan, with discussion of receptor binding, downstream effects, side-effect (vs ACE inhibitors). You could frame a case: "50 yo male with hypertension cannot tolerate ACE inhibitor cough; switched to losartan (AT_1R antagonist) …" and show receptor pharmacology.

Citation:Sica DA. Pharmacology and clinical efficacy of angiotensin receptor blockers. Am J Hypertens. 2001 Aug;14(4 Suppl 1):242S-247S. doi:10.1016/S0895-7061(01)02134-3. OUP Academic

CHAPTER 6

APELIN RECEPTORS

Apelin receptors, also known as APJ receptors, are G-protein-coupled receptors (GPCRs) activated by the endogenous ligands apelin and elabela (also known as toddler). These receptors are involved in regulating cardiovascular functions, fluid homeostasis, and energy metabolism. They play a critical role in various physiological and pathological processes.

Definition of Apelin Receptors

The apelin receptor is a GPCR encoded by the APLNR gene. It binds to apelin, a peptide derived from preproapelin, as well as elabela, another peptide ligand. Apelin receptors share structural similarity with angiotensin II type 1 receptors but function independently of angiotensin II.

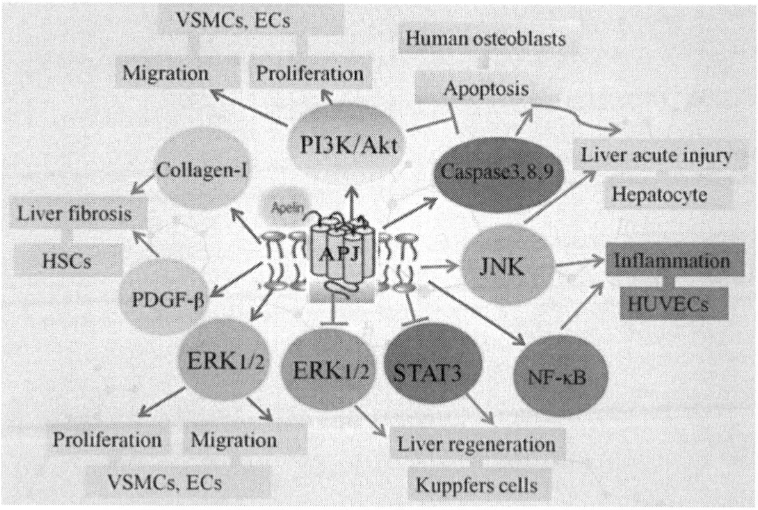

Fig. 5.1 Apelin receptors and activation.

Classification

Unlike other GPCR families, apelin receptors are not divided into subtypes. The single receptor type has multiple endogenous ligands, primarily apelin and elabela, which can modulate its activity depending on the physiological context.

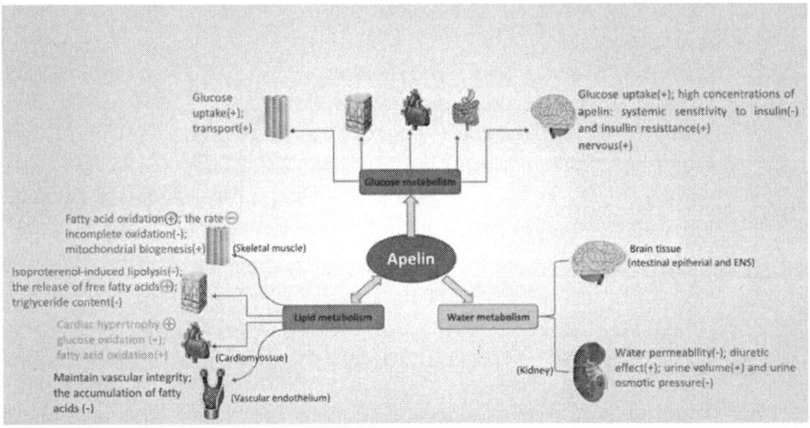

Fig. 5.2 Physilogical actions of Apelin receptors.

Pharmacological Actions

1. **Cardiovascular Effects**:
    - **Vasodilation**: it enhances nitric oxide (NO) production, reducing vascular resistance.
    - **Inotropic Effects**: it improves cardiac contractility, reducing preload and afterload.
    - **Anti-hypertensive Actions**: it Lowers blood pressure through vasodilation and renal effects.
2. **Fluid and Electrolyte Homeostasis**:
    - It Modulates vasopressin release, influencing water retention.
    - It Promotes natriuresis and diuresis through renal mechanisms.
3. **Energy Metabolism**:
    - It Regulates glucose uptake and insulin sensitivity.
    - It Modulates lipid metabolism and fat storage.
4. **Angiogenesis**: It Stimulates blood vessel formation and promotes endothelial cell proliferation.

5. **Anti-fibrotic Effects**: It Reduces cardiac and renal fibrosis in pathological states.

Indications of Apelin Receptor Modulation

1. **Heart Failure**: Apelinanalogs improve myocardial contractility and reduce vascular resistance, making them beneficial in heart failure treatment.
2. **Pulmonary Arterial Hypertension (PAH)**: Reduces pulmonary vascular resistance and vascular remodeling.
3. **Ischemic Heart Disease**: Enhances coronary blood flow and limits ischemia-reperfusion injury.
4. **Metabolic Disorders**: A potential therapeutic target for obesity, type 2 diabetes, and metabolic syndrome.
5. **Kidney Diseases**: Protects against ischemic injury and supports renal blood flow regulation.

Contraindications

1. **Hypotension**: Apelin receptor agonists can exacerbate low blood pressure due to their vasodilatory effects.
2. **Severe Cardiovascular Dysfunction**: Its Overactivation may worsen conditions with impaired myocardial contractility or vascular tone regulation.
3. **Pregnancy**: Limited data on safety; use in pregnancy is generally avoided unless benefits outweigh risks.
4. **Severe Renal or Hepatic Impairment**: Altered pharmacokinetics may increase the risk of adverse effects in these populations.

CHAPTER 7

BILE ACID RECEPTORS

Bile acid receptors are a group of nuclear and membrane-bound receptors that regulate various metabolic processes, including bile acid homeostasis, lipid metabolism, glucose regulation, and inflammatory responses. These receptors play a pivotal role in maintaining metabolic and digestive health.

Definition of Bile Acid Receptors

Bile acid receptors are specialized proteins that bind bile acids as ligands to mediate their effects on cellular and systemic physiology. They act as sensors for bile acid concentrations and orchestrate downstream signaling to maintain metabolic balance.

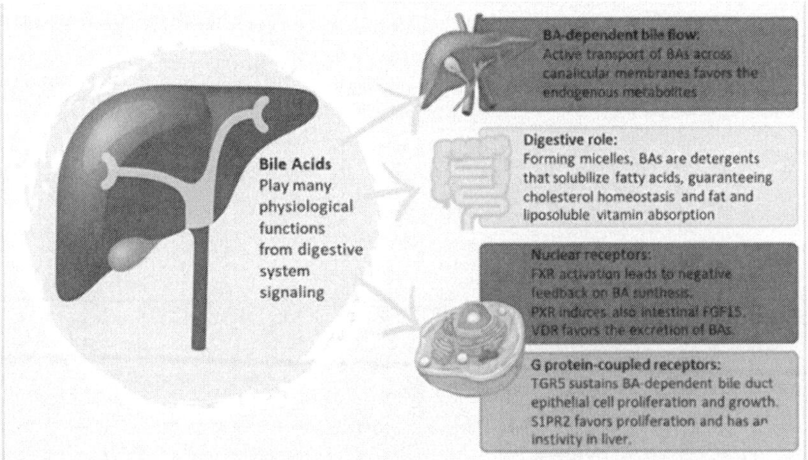

Fig. 6.1 Bile release and physiological actions in human body.

Table 6.1 Classification of bile receptors, diffrenr ligands, locations and functions of its types.

ReceptRe ceptor	**Representatrepr esentative Ligands**	**Cytogeccy togenetic Location**	**Tissue/Cell Expression**	**Functions**
FXR (NR1H4)	CDCA > DCA > LCA > CA; INT-747, GW4064, fexaramine, PX-102	12q23.1	Liver, intestine, kidney, adrenal gland	• Bile acid metabolism • Glucose metabolism • Lipid metabolism • Liver regeneration • Anti-inflammatory
VDR (NR1I1)	LCA; Vitamin D; LY2108491	12q13.11	Liver, intestine, gallbladder, bone, kidney, parathyroid, skin, bone marrow	• Bile acid synthesis • Xenobiotic detoxification • Calcium homeostasis • Antimicrobial defense
PXR (NR1I2)	LCA, DCA, CA; progesterone; rifampicin	3q13.33	Liver, intestine, immune cells	• Bile acid synthesis • Glucose metabolism • Lipid metabolism • Drug metabolism • Anti-inflammatory
CAR (NR1I3)	CA, 6-keto-LCA, 12-keto-LCA; phenobarbital	1q23.3	Liver, intestine, kidney	• Xenobiotic detoxification • Glucose metabolism • Lipid metabolism
TGR5	LCA > DCA > CDCA > CA; INT-767; oleanolic acid	2q35	Liver, intestine, gallbladder, muscle, brown adipose, brain	• Glucose homeostasis • Intestinal motility • Gallbladder relaxation •

				Energy metabolism • Anti-inflammatory

Classification of Bile Acid Receptors

Bile acid receptors are classified into two major types:

1. **Nuclear Receptors**:
   - **Farnesoid X Receptor (FXR)**: A key regulator of bile acid synthesis and metabolism. FXR is activated by bile acids such as chenodeoxycholic acid.
2. **Membrane-Bound Receptors**:
   - **TGR5 (G-protein-coupled bile acid receptor 1)**: A GPCR involved in energy metabolism, anti-inflammatory pathways, and gut hormone regulation.

Pharmacological Actions of Bile Acid Receptors

1. **Farnesoid X Receptor (FXR)**: Its stimulation includes
   - **Regulation of Bile Acid Homeostasis**: Suppresses bile acid synthesis by inhibiting CYP7A1, the rate-limiting enzyme in bile acid production.
   - **Lipid Metabolism**: Reduces triglyceride synthesis and promotes cholesterol elimination.
   - **Anti-inflammatory Actions**: Inhibits pro-inflammatory cytokines and protects against liver and intestinal inflammation.
   - **Glucose Regulation**: Enhances insulin sensitivity and reduces hepatic glucose production.
2. **TGR5**: Its stimulation includes
   - **Energy Expenditure**: Promotes thermogenesis in brown adipose tissue and skeletal muscle.
   - **Gut Hormone Secretion**: Stimulates GLP-1 release, enhancing glucose metabolism and insulin secretion.
   - **Anti-inflammatory Effects**: Reduces inflammation by suppressing macrophage activation and cytokine release.

Indications of Bile Acid Receptor Modulation

1. **Cholestatic Liver Diseases**: FXR agonists like obeticholic acid are used to treat primary biliary cholangitis and other cholestatic conditions by reducing bile acid toxicity.
2. **Non-Alcoholic Fatty Liver Disease (NAFLD) and Non-Alcoholic Steatohepatitis (NASH)**: FXR activation improves lipid metabolism and reduces hepatic inflammation and fibrosis.
3. **Metabolic Disorders**: TGR5 agonists are potential treatments for obesity, type 2 diabetes, and metabolic syndrome due to their effects on glucose and energy homeostasis.
4. **Inflammatory Bowel Disease (IBD)**: Bile acid receptor modulation reduces intestinal inflammation and enhances mucosal repair.
5. **Hyperlipidemia**: FXR activation lowers triglycerides and improves cholesterol profiles.

Contraindications of Bile Acid Receptor Modulation

1. **Severe Hepatic Impairment**: FXR agonists may exacerbate liver dysfunction in patients with advanced liver disease.
2. **Gallbladder Disorders**: Increased bile flow due to TGR5 activation may promote gallstone formation in susceptible individuals.
3. **Pregnancy and Lactation**: Limited safety data; bile acid receptor modulators should be used with caution during pregnancy and breastfeeding.
4. **Severe Renal Impairment**: Altered drug clearance may lead to adverse effects, necessitating dose adjustments or avoidance.

CHAPTER 8

BOMBESIN RECEPTORS

Bombesin receptors are a class of G protein-coupled receptors (GPCRs) that are activated by bombesin-like peptides. These receptors are involved in regulating a variety of physiological processes, including gastrointestinal function, secretion of hormones, and neural activity.

1. Definition of Bombesin Receptors

Bombesin receptors are a group of receptors that respond to bombesin, a peptide found in amphibians. Bombesin and its analogs, such as neuromedin B and gastrin-releasing peptide (GRP), are endogenous ligands for these receptors. These receptors are implicated in several biological processes like regulating gastric secretion, neuropeptide signaling, and cellular proliferation.

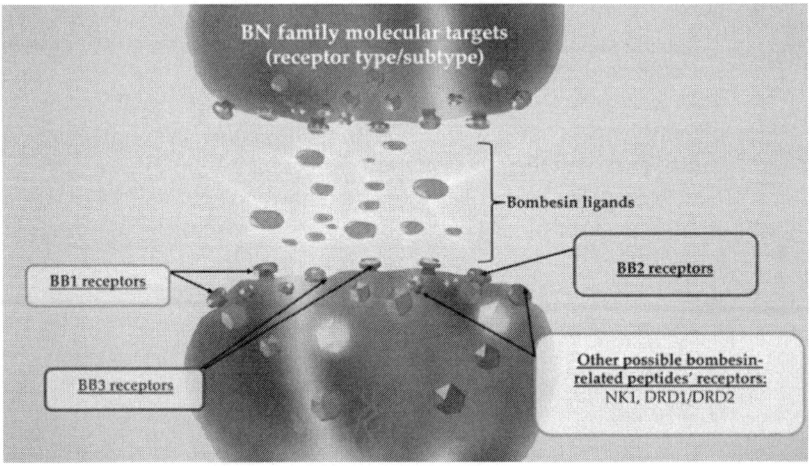

Fig 8.1 Types of Bombesin receptors.

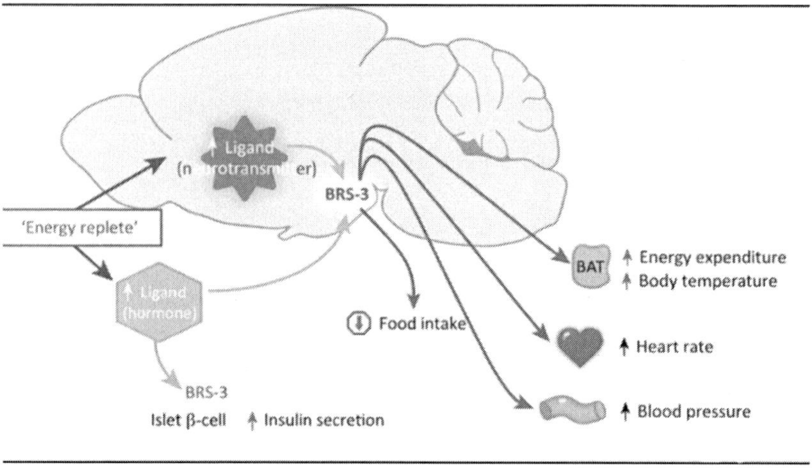

Fig 8.2 binding of ligands with BRS-3 receptors and pharmacological actions.

2. Classification of Bombesin Receptors

Bombesin receptors can be classified into four subtypes based on the ligand specificity and distribution in tissues:

- **BB1 Receptor (GRP receptor)**: Primarily binds to gastrin-releasing peptide (GRP), involved in the regulation of gastric secretion and smooth muscle activity.
- **BB2 Receptor (Neuromedin B receptor)**: Binds to neuromedin B, playing roles in neuroendocrine function, smooth muscle contraction, and thermoregulation.
- **BB3 Receptor**: Primarily binds to bombesin itself, and its function is more closely associated with processes such as appetite regulation and thermogenesis.
- **BB4 Receptor**: This receptor is less well-characterized, and its physiological role remains under investigation.

3. Pharmacological Actions

Bombesin receptors mediate various pharmacological actions through different signaling pathways. Some of the major effects include:

- **Gastric Secretion and Digestive Function**: Activation of bombesin receptors in the gastrointestinal tract can stimulate the release of gastric acid and digestive enzymes, aiding digestion.
- **Smooth Muscle Contraction**: Bombesin receptor activation can cause smooth muscle contraction in various organs, including the stomach and intestines.
- **Neuroendocrine Regulation**: Bombesin receptors are involved in the regulation of hormone release, including prolactin, insulin, and growth hormone, which play significant roles in growth, metabolism, and reproductive functions.
- **Thermoregulation**: In the hypothalamus, bombesin receptors contribute to the regulation of body temperature by affecting heat production and energy expenditure.
- **Cellular Proliferation**: Bombesin receptors are involved in the regulation of cell growth and differentiation, making them relevant in cancer biology, particularly in certain types of neuroendocrine tumors.

4. Indications for Use

Bombesin receptor agonists or antagonists are studied for their therapeutic potential in various clinical areas:

- **Cancer Treatment**: Bombesin receptors, particularly BB2 and BB3, are expressed in various tumors, including neuroendocrine cancers, breast cancer, and prostate cancer. Targeting bombesin receptors with radiolabeled peptides has shown promise in tumor imaging and therapy.
- **Gastrointestinal Disorders**: Drugs targeting bombesin receptors may be used to manage conditions like irritable bowel syndrome (IBS) or functional dyspepsia, where bombesin signaling may be dysregulated.
- **Obesity and Metabolic Disorders**: Because bombesin receptors are involved in regulating appetite and metabolism, they may have potential in treating obesity and other metabolic disorders.
- **Pain and Neurological Disorders**: Bombesin receptors in the central nervous system may be targeted to modulate pain perception and other neurological conditions.

5. Contraindications

The use of bombesin receptor-based drugs or therapies may be contraindicated in certain conditions, including:

- **Pregnancy and Breastfeeding**: The effects of bombesin receptor modulation during pregnancy and lactation are not well established, so caution is advised.
- **Cancer**: In cases where tumors overexpress bombesin receptors, therapies that target these receptors may not be recommended if the tumor type or location has adverse reactions to the treatment.
- **Hypersensitivity to Bombesin**: Individuals with known hypersensitivity to bombesin peptides or analogs may be at risk for allergic reactions or other adverse effects.
- **Cardiovascular Disorders**: As bombesin receptor activation can affect smooth muscle and blood vessels, individuals with certain cardiovascular conditions may experience adverse effects, such as hypertension or arrhythmias.

CHAPTER 9

BRADYKININ RECEPTORS

Bradykinin receptors are G-protein-coupled receptors (GPCRs) that are activated by bradykinin, a peptide that plays a central role in inflammation, blood pressure regulation, pain perception, and vasodilation. Bradykinin is a key mediator in the kinin-kallikrein system, and it exerts its biological effects by binding to two main receptor types: B1 receptors and B2 receptors.

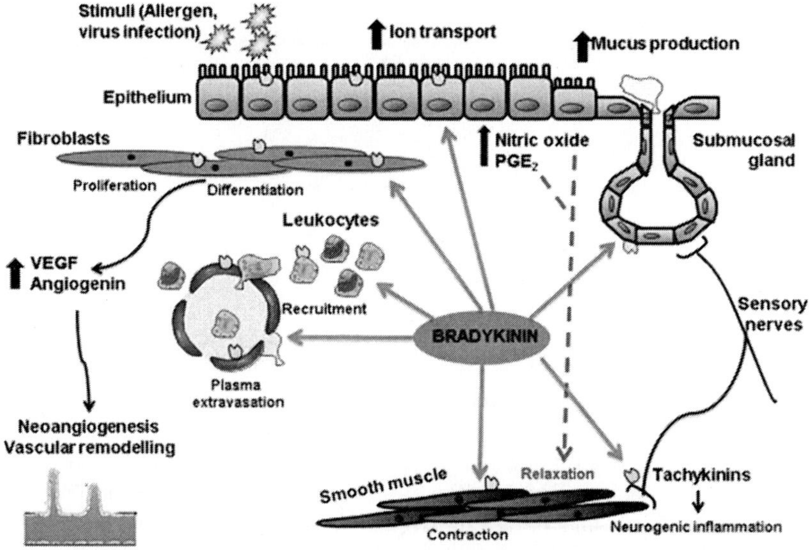

Fig 9.1 Bradykinin receptors and pharmacological actions at different site of the body.

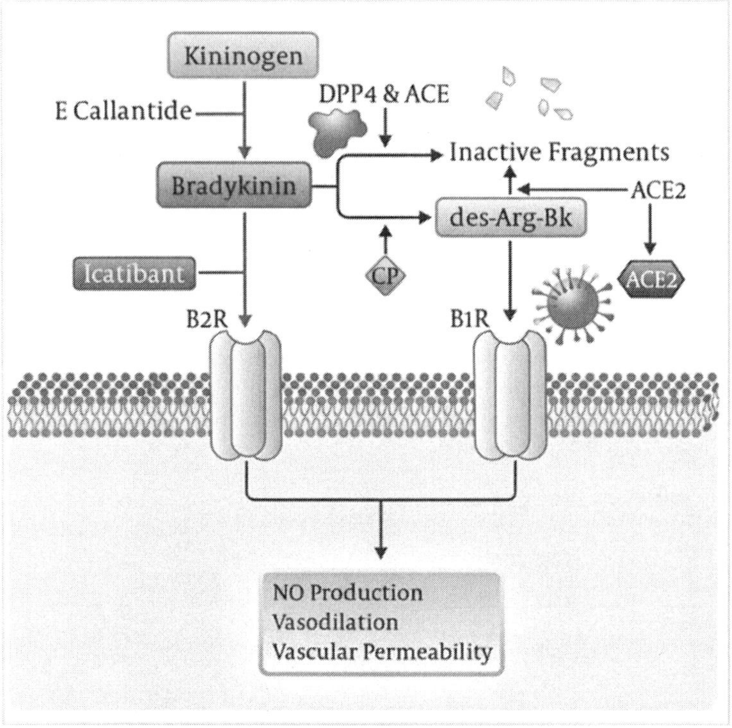

Fig 9.2 Bradkinin binding with receptors and pharmacological actions.

2. Classification of Bradykinin Receptors

Bradykinin receptors are classified into two subtypes based on their ligand specificity and functional roles:

- **B2 Receptor (BK2R)**: The B2 receptor is the primary receptor for bradykinin and is constitutively expressed in a variety of tissues, including vascular smooth muscle, endothelial cells, and kidneys. It mediates most of the classical actions of bradykinin, such as vasodilation, increased vascular permeability, and pain.
- **B1 Receptor (BK1R)**: The B1 receptor is typically not expressed under normal conditions but is induced by tissue injury, inflammation, or chronic conditions such as arthritis. It is primarily involved in the inflammatory response and can contribute to pain and tissue damage when activated.

3. Pharmacological Actions of Bradykinin Receptors

The activation of bradykinin receptors leads to a variety of biological effects through different signaling pathways:

B2 Receptor Actions:

- **Vasodilation**: The activation of the B2 receptor leads to the release of nitric oxide (NO) and prostacyclin, which promote vasodilation and reduce blood pressure.
- **Increased Vascular Permeability**: Bradykinin binding to B2 receptors causes endothelial cell contraction and increases the permeability of blood vessels, leading to the extravasation of fluids and proteins, contributing to inflammation and edema.
- **Pain and Sensory Nerve Stimulation**: Bradykinin activates sensory nerve endings, contributing to pain, particularly in inflammatory conditions like arthritis.
- **Smooth Muscle Contraction**: It can induce smooth muscle contraction, particularly in the gastrointestinal and respiratory tracts, and plays a role in airway constriction during allergic reactions.
- **Renal Effects**: Bradykinin can affect kidney function, influencing sodium balance and fluid regulation.

B1 Receptor Actions: its stimulatrory effects includes

- **Inflammation**: B1 receptor activation plays a role in chronic inflammation and can exacerbate inflammatory conditions like rheumatoid arthritis. It promotes the release of pro-inflammatory cytokines, further amplifying the inflammatory response.
- **Pain**: The B1 receptor is involved in inflammatory pain pathways, especially during tissue injury or inflammation.
- **Vasodilation**: Similar to B2 receptor activation, B1 receptor activation can also promote vasodilation, although this is generally a secondary effect related to inflammation.

4. Indications for Use

Due to their involvement in a variety of physiological and pathological processes, bradykinin receptors have therapeutic potential in several clinical areas:

- **Hypertension**: Bradykinin's vasodilatory effect via the B2 receptor contributes to blood pressure regulation, making bradykinin receptor modulators useful in controlling hypertension.
- **Angioedema**: B2 receptor antagonists or inhibitors are studied for their role in treating hereditary or acquired angioedema, a condition where bradykinin-induced vasodilation and vascular permeability lead to edema (swelling), particularly in the face, airway, and extremities.
- **Pain Management**: Given bradykinin's role in pain perception, both B1 and B2 receptor antagonists are being explored for managing pain, particularly in inflammatory pain and conditions like osteoarthritis and rheumatoid arthritis.
- **Chronic Inflammation**: B1 receptor antagonists may help in treating chronic inflammatory diseases by reducing inflammation and pain associated with conditions like arthritis.
- **Cardiovascular Diseases**: Bradykinin's effects on blood vessels, particularly its role in vasodilation, are being investigated for their potential benefits in treating cardiovascular diseases like coronary artery disease, heart failure, and myocardial infarction.
- **Renal Protection**: Given bradykinin's role in renal function, certain receptor modulators are studied for their protective effects on kidneys in conditions such as diabetic nephropathy.

5. Contraindications

Bradykinin receptor antagonists or agonists should be used with caution or avoided in the following conditions:

- **Pregnancy and Lactation**: The use of bradykinin receptor modulators in pregnancy and lactation should be avoided unless clearly necessary, as their effects on fetal development and milk production are not fully understood. In particular, bradykinin can contribute to changes in vascular tone, which might pose risks in pregnancy.
- **Hypersensitivity to Bradykinin**: People with hypersensitivity to bradykinin or its analogs should avoid drugs that interact with bradykinin receptors due to the risk of allergic reactions, including anaphylaxis.
- **Angioedema or History of Angioedema**: Patients with a history of bradykinin-mediated angioedema, especially hereditary angioedema, should avoid drugs that increase bradykinin levels

(such as ACE inhibitors or bradykinin receptor antagonists) as this can precipitate episodes of severe swelling, particularly in the airway.

- **Renal Impairment**: While bradykinin's role in kidney function is complex, caution should be exercised when using bradykinin receptor modulators in patients with severe renal impairment due to potential alterations in fluid and electrolyte balance.
- **Low Blood Pressure (Hypotension)**: Bradykinin's vasodilatory effects can lower blood pressure. Therefore, drugs targeting bradykinin receptors should be avoided or used cautiously in individuals with hypotension or those at risk for low blood pressure.

CHAPTER 10

CALCITONIN RECEPTORS

Calcitonin receptors are G-protein-coupled receptors (GPCRs) that mediate the biological effects of calcitonin, a hormone primarily involved in calcium and bone metabolism. Calcitonin is produced by the parafollicular cells (C cells) of the thyroid gland. When it binds to its receptors, calcitonin exerts a variety of effects, particularly in regulating blood calcium levels, promoting bone health, and influencing calcium homeostasis. There are two primary receptor subtypes: calcitonin receptor (CTR) and calcitonin gene-related peptide receptor (CGRP receptor).

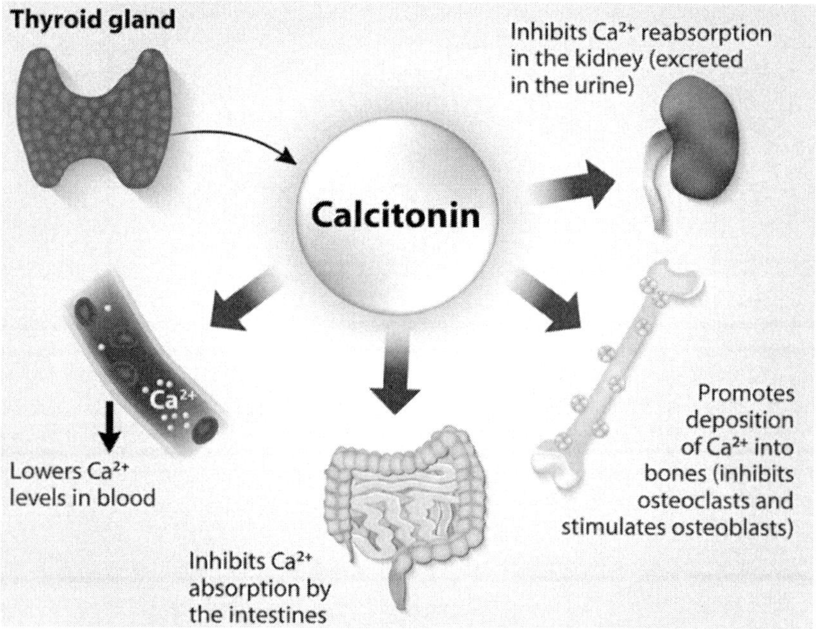

Fig 10.1 the effect of calcitonin in human body.

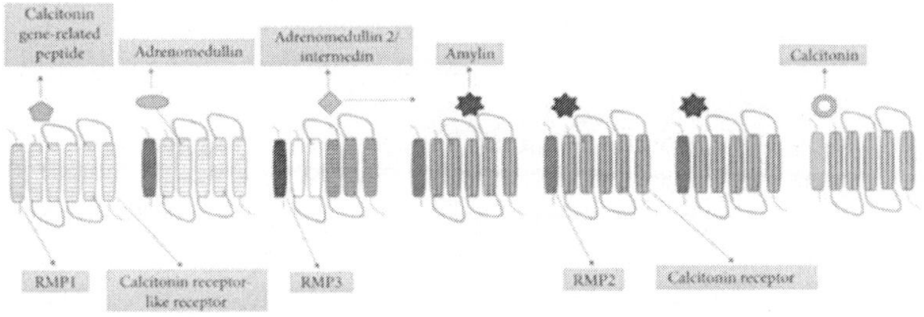

Fig. 10.2 Different ligans and their binding with calcitonin receptors

2. Classification of Calcitonin Receptors

Calcitonin receptors can be classified as follows:

- **Calcitonin Receptor (CTR)**: This is the primary receptor for calcitonin. It is widely distributed in various tissues, including the bones, kidneys, and brain. It plays a significant role in regulating calcium homeostasis and bone metabolism by mediating the actions of calcitonin.
- **Calcitonin Gene-Related Peptide (CGRP) Receptor**: This receptor, while primarily involved in the effects of calcitonin gene-related peptide (CGRP), can also interact with calcitonin, although its primary function is related to vasodilation and modulation of neurotransmission. This receptor is expressed in the central nervous system and peripheral tissues, including smooth muscle.

3. Pharmacological Actions of Calcitonin Receptors

The activation of calcitonin receptors leads to several important biological actions, primarily concerning calcium metabolism and bone regulation:

Calcitonin Receptor (CTR) Actions:

- **Inhibition of Osteoclast Activity**: Calcitonin binding to its receptor on osteoclasts (bone-resorbing cells) inhibits their activity, leading to decreased bone resorption and a net increase in bone mass. This effect is important in preventing excessive calcium release from bones into the bloodstream.

- **Reduction of Serum Calcium Levels**: By inhibiting osteoclast activity and reducing the release of calcium from bones, calcitonin helps lower blood calcium levels, particularly in conditions like hypercalcemia.
- **Kidney Function**: Calcitonin has renal actions, including reducing renal tubular reabsorption of calcium and phosphate, leading to their excretion in urine. This further helps in regulating blood calcium levels.
- **Pain Modulation**: Calcitonin may influence pain perception, particularly in conditions associated with bone loss or fractures. It has been shown to have analgesic effects, likely due to its ability to inhibit osteoclast-mediated bone resorption.

Calcitonin Gene-Related Peptide (CGRP) Receptor Actions:

- **Vasodilation**: CGRP receptors, activated by CGRP (a neuropeptide), mediate vasodilation, contributing to increased blood flow. Though calcitonin does not primarily mediate this effect, its interaction with CGRP receptors can influence vascular tone.
- **Neurotransmission and Pain**: CGRP receptors are involved in pain transmission and neurogenic inflammation, particularly in the context of migraine and other neurological conditions. However, calcitonin's effect on CGRP receptors is secondary to its role on CTR.

4. Indications for Use

Calcitonin receptor agonists (such as synthetic or recombinant calcitonin) and antagonists are used in various clinical settings:

- **Hypercalcemia**: Calcitonin is used in the treatment of hypercalcemia (elevated blood calcium levels), particularly in malignancy-associated hypercalcemia, where it helps lower serum calcium levels by inhibiting osteoclast activity and enhancing renal calcium excretion.
- **Osteoporosis**: Calcitonin is used to treat osteoporosis, especially in postmenopausal women or individuals with Paget's disease. It works by inhibiting bone resorption and promoting bone density, reducing the risk of fractures.

- **Paget's disease of Bone**: Calcitonin is employed in the treatment of Paget's disease, a condition characterized by excessive bone resorption and abnormal bone remodeling. The hormone helps normalize bone turnover and relieve pain.
- **Bone Pain**: Calcitonin is used as a part of pain management, particularly in bone pain resulting from conditions like vertebral fractures or metastatic bone disease. Its ability to inhibit bone resorption and osteoclast activity may help relieve pain in such cases.
- **Acute Vertebral Compression Fractures**: Calcitonin may be administered to alleviate pain and reduce the risk of further complications in patients suffering from acute vertebral compression fractures due to osteoporosis.
- **Migraine Treatment**: Although not a primary indication for calcitonin itself, the CGRP receptor interaction is a target for certain migraine therapies. CGRP receptor antagonists are being developed for migraine treatment, utilizing the vasodilation and pain modulation properties of CGRP.

5. Contraindications

The use of calcitonin receptor-based therapies may be contraindicated in certain conditions:

- **Hypersensitivity to Calcitonin**: Individuals with a known hypersensitivity or allergy to calcitonin or its components should avoid calcitonin-based treatments due to the risk of allergic reactions, including anaphylaxis.
- **Renal Impairment**: While calcitonin has effects on renal function, particularly in increasing the excretion of calcium and phosphate, its use in patients with significant renal impairment should be cautious. In such cases, close monitoring of renal function is necessary.
- **Pregnancy and Lactation**: The use of calcitonin during pregnancy is generally not recommended unless the benefits outweigh the risks, as the effects on fetal development are not fully established. Calcitonin is also excreted in breast milk, so caution is advised when administering it to breastfeeding mothers.
- **Hypocalcemia**: Although calcitonin is used to lower calcium levels in hypercalcemia, it may exacerbate hypocalcemia (low calcium levels) and should not be used in patients with this condition.

- **Bone Marrow Disorders**: Caution is required in patients with bone marrow disorders, such as leukemia or lymphoma, as the inhibitory effects of calcitonin on osteoclasts may interfere with bone marrow function or affect bone metabolism in these conditions.

CHAPTER 11

CALCIUM-SENSING RECEPTORS (CASR)

Calcium-sensing receptors (CaSR) are G-protein-coupled receptors (GPCRs) that play a critical role in maintaining calcium homeostasis in the body. These receptors are primarily found in the parathyroid glands, kidneys, bones, and gastrointestinal tract. CaSR is highly sensitive to extracellular calcium levels and regulates the secretion of parathyroid hormone (PTH) and various physiological processes involved in calcium and phosphate balance. It ensures that blood calcium levels are kept within a narrow, optimal range, which is essential for various cellular and metabolic functions.

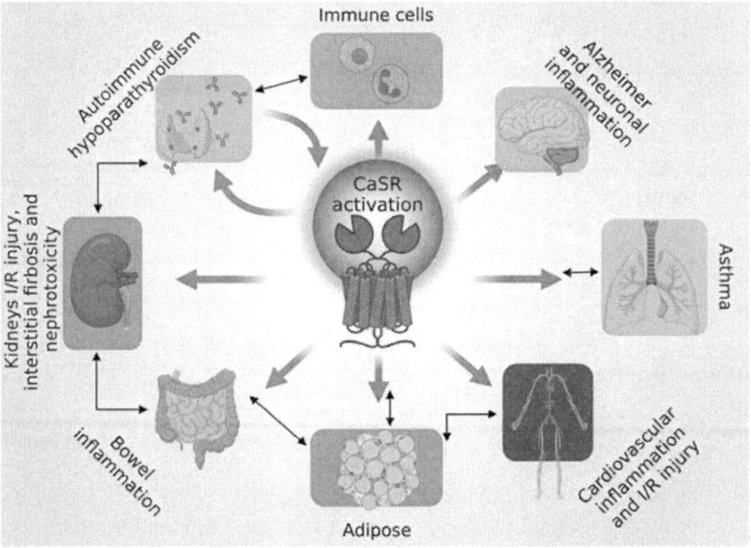

Fig. 11.1 different actions produced by calcium sensing receptors.

2. Classification of Calcium-Sensing Receptors

CaSR is a single receptor but can exhibit different behaviors and effects depending on the tissue and the type of ligand that activates it. There are no formal subtypes in the same way as other receptors, but the receptor can interact with various ligands:

- **Endogenous Agonists**: The primary endogenous ligand for CaSRis extracellular calcium. Other activators include magnesium (in certain contexts) and certain amino acids.
- **Antagonists and Agonists**: The CaSR can also be modulated by synthetic compounds, including small molecule agonists and antagonists, which are being researched for therapeutic use.

3. Pharmacological Actions of Calcium-Sensing Receptors

The activation of CaSR leads to various cellular responses through different signaling pathways. The pharmacological actions of CaSR are largely focused on the regulation of calcium and phosphate balance and are crucial for multiple physiological processes:

Regulation of Parathyroid Hormone (PTH) Secretion:

- **Inhibition of PTH Secretion**: When CaSR is activated by increased levels of extracellular calcium, it inhibits the release of parathyroid hormone (PTH) from the parathyroid glands. PTH is a key hormone that regulates calcium homeostasis. By inhibiting PTH secretion, CaSR helps reduce calcium release from bones and decrease renal calcium reabsorption, thus lowering blood calcium levels.

Kidney Function:

- **Regulation of Renal Calcium Reabsorption**: CaSR plays a significant role in regulating calcium reabsorption in the kidneys. In response to high calcium levels, the receptor reduces calcium reabsorption, which leads to increased calcium excretion in urine. Conversely, under low calcium conditions, it enhances calcium reabsorption to conserve calcium.

Bone Remodeling:

- **Bone Resorption Regulation**: CaSR is involved in the regulation of bone remodeling by influencing osteoclast activity. When activated by high calcium levels, it can inhibit osteoclast-mediated bone resorption, helping to prevent excessive bone loss. On the other hand, reduced calcium levels may stimulate bone resorption.

Gastrointestinal System:

- **Modulation of Calcium Absorption**: In the gastrointestinal tract, CaSR influences calcium absorption by regulating the function of the enterocytes (cells lining the intestines). In response to low extracellular calcium, it increases the expression of calcium transporters to enhance calcium absorption.

Parathyroid Cells and Hormone Secretion:

- **Intracellular Signaling**: The activation of CaSR triggers several intracellular signaling pathways, including those involving phospholipase C, protein kinase C, and intracellular calcium mobilization, which mediate the effects on PTH secretion, renal calcium handling, and bone resorption.

4. Indications for Use

CaSR modulators (both agonists and antagonists) have therapeutic potential in various medical conditions related to calcium imbalance. These include:

- **Hypercalcemia**: Calcium-sensing receptor agonists are being explored to treat conditions characterized by elevated calcium levels, such as in **primary hyperparathyroidism** or **hypercalcemia of malignancy**. By increasing CaSR activation, they may help decrease PTH secretion and lower calcium levels.
- **Hypocalcemia**: On the flip side, calcium-sensing receptor antagonists could be used to treat hypocalcemia (low blood calcium levels), particularly in conditions such as **hypoparathyroidism**, where there is insufficient PTH secretion. These antagonists may help increase calcium reabsorption and PTH secretion, thus increasing calcium levels in the blood.

- **Chronic Kidney Disease (CKD)**: In CKD, CaSR is involved in the dysregulation of calcium and phosphate balance, leading to conditions such as secondary hyperparathyroidism and ectopic calcification. CaSR modulators are being researched to restore calcium balance and improve kidney function by modulating PTH secretion and calcium metabolism.
- **Osteoporosis**: Because CaSR regulates bone remodeling, researchers are investigating CaSR modulators to improve bone density in diseases like osteoporosis by reducing excessive bone resorption.
- **Nephrolithiasis (Kidney Stones)**: Since CaSR is involved in calcium regulation by the kidneys, CaSR agonists could be explored to help prevent calcium-based kidney stones by reducing calcium excretion.
- **Paget's Disease of Bone**: In Paget's disease, CaSR modulation may help prevent excessive bone resorption and abnormal bone remodeling by osteoclasts.

5. Contraindications

While CaSR modulators may be beneficial for certain medical conditions, there are several potential contraindications to their use:

- **Hypercalcemia**: Use of CaSR agonists may be contraindicated in patients with hypercalcemia due to increased risk of exacerbating the condition. Excessive activation of the receptor can further suppress PTH secretion, worsening calcium imbalance in certain contexts.
- **Severe Renal Impairment**: Patients with significant kidney dysfunction may experience altered calcium handling, and the use of CaSR modulators should be carefully monitored in such cases. In some instances, the modulation of renal calcium reabsorption may be inappropriate, particularly in patients with end-stage renal disease.
- **Hypocalcemia**: The use of CaSR antagonists in hypocalcemic patients (such as those with hypoparathyroidism) should be avoided unless under strict medical supervision, as it may worsen the calcium deficiency.
- **Pregnancy and Lactation**: The use of CaSR modulators in pregnant or breastfeeding women should be approached with

caution, as the effects of these drugs on fetal development and milk production are not fully understood.

- **Hyperparathyroidism**: Caution is advised when using CaSR agonists in cases of secondary hyperparathyroidism (particularly in patients with chronic kidney disease), as they could potentially exacerbate underlying calcium and phosphate imbalances.
- **Bone Disorders**: Since CaSR is involved in bone resorption, caution should be exercised in patients with metabolic bone diseases (e.g., osteogenesis imperfecta) or patients at risk for osteoporosis, as modulating CaSR activity may impact bone health.

Clinical Importance

L-type calcium channels — CCB (amlodipine)-induced vasodilation and overdose management

Vignette idea: Hypertensive patient started on amlodipine develops marked peripheral edema and hypotension after an accidental extra dose; explain L-type Ca^{2+} channel blockade in vascular smooth muscle and cardiovascular adverse effects (and overdose therapy).

Reference/Review (pharmacology and clinical): standard pharmacology texts and CCB overdose reviews (you can pair with clinical case reports in emergency medicine literature).

CHAPTER 12

CANNABINOID RECEPTORS

Cannabinoid receptors are a type of G-protein-coupled receptor (GPCR) that mediate the effects of cannabinoids, the active compounds in cannabis (marijuana), as well as synthetic cannabinoids.

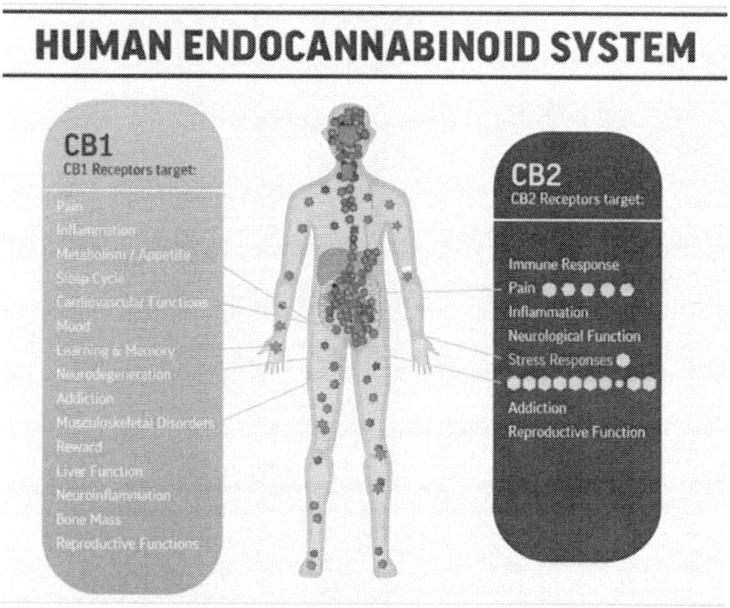

Fig. 12.1 different types of endocannabinoid receptors and pharmacological actions in human body.

These receptors are involved in a wide range of physiological processes, including pain modulation, appetite regulation, mood, and memory. The two primary cannabinoid receptor types are:

- **CB1 Receptors**: Predominantly found in the central nervous system (CNS), particularly in the brain, spinal cord, and peripheral nervous system. They are involved in mediating the psychoactive effects of cannabinoids, such as those produced by tetrahydrocannabinol (THC).
- **CB2 Receptors**: Mainly found in immune cells and tissues, such as the spleen, tonsils, and other peripheral organs. They are involved in immune system modulation and are less associated with the psychoactive effects seen with CB1 activation.

2. Classification of Cannabinoid Receptors

Cannabinoid receptors are classified into two main types, each with distinct locations and roles:

- **CB1 Receptor**: **Location**: Primarily located in the brain (especially the hippocampus, cortex, and basal ganglia), spinal cord, and peripheral nervous system.
  Function: Regulates neurotransmitter release and plays a significant role in mood, memory, motor function, and pain perception. It is primarily responsible for the psychoactive effects of cannabis.
- **CB2 Receptor**: **Location**: Primarily located in peripheral tissues, such as the immune system (including the spleen and lymph nodes), gastrointestinal tract, and peripheral nervous system.
  Function: Modulates immune responses, inflammation, and pain sensation, with potential therapeutic implications for conditions involving inflammation, immune modulation, and tissue repair.

3. Pharmacological Actions of Cannabinoid Receptors

The pharmacological effects of cannabinoid receptors arise from their activation by endogenous cannabinoids (endocannabinoids), plant-derived cannabinoids (e.g., THC), and synthetic cannabinoids. The actions of these receptors differ based on the type of receptor and its location in the body.

CB1 Receptor Pharmacological Actions:

1. **Psychoactive Effects**: CB1 receptor activation by THC, the main psychoactive compound in cannabis, produces feelings of euphoria,

altered sensory perception, and changes in mood. This is why THC is associated with the "high" experienced by cannabis users.

2. **Pain Modulation**: CB1 receptors play a significant role in the modulation of pain, particularly in the CNS. Activation of CB1 receptors in areas of the brain and spinal cord can reduce the perception of pain.
3. **Appetite Stimulation**: CB1 receptor activation is involved in increasing appetite and promoting food intake, which is why cannabinoids (such as THC) are used therapeutically to help stimulate appetite in conditions like cancer, HIV/AIDS, and anorexia.
4. **Cognitive and Memory Effects**: CB1 receptors are involved in cognitive processes like learning and memory. Their activation can impair short-term memory, coordination, and concentration, which is commonly associated with cannabis use.
5. **Motor Control**: CB1 receptors in the basal ganglia regulate motor function. Activation can lead to motor impairments, such as tremors or coordination problems.

CB2 Receptor Pharmacological Actions:

1. **Anti-Inflammatory Effects**: CB2 receptors are predominantly found in immune cells, and their activation is associated with the modulation of immune responses and inflammation. By reducing the release of pro-inflammatory cytokines, CB2 receptor activation can have therapeutic effects in conditions like rheumatoid arthritis and inflammatory bowel disease.
2. **Pain Relief**: CB2 receptors can also modulate peripheral pain by interacting with pain receptors in tissues outside the CNS. They can be involved in reducing pain in inflammatory conditions.
3. **Neuroprotection**: While CB2 receptors are less involved in cognitive processes, their activation may have neuroprotective effects, helping protect neurons from oxidative stress and inflammation, which could be useful in neurodegenerative diseases like Alzheimer's and Parkinson's.
4. **Immune System Modulation**: CB2 receptors play a role in modulating the activity of various immune cells, such as macrophages and T cells, helping control the immune response and inflammation.

4. Indications for Use

Cannabinoid receptor modulators (agonists or antagonists) have potential therapeutic uses in various conditions:

CB1 Receptor Agonists (e.g., THC):

1. **Pain Management**: THC is used in managing chronic pain, particularly in conditions like neuropathic pain, cancer-related pain, and multiple sclerosis (MS). It works by reducing pain perception in the CNS.
2. **Appetite Stimulation**: THC and synthetic cannabinoids are used to treat appetite loss, particularly in cancer patients undergoing chemotherapy, those with HIV/AIDS, and individuals with anorexia.
3. **Neurological Disorders**: THC and other CB1 agonists are being explored for their potential benefits in managing symptoms of neurological diseases such as MS, epilepsy, and Parkinson's disease. Their effects on spasticity, tremors, and seizures may help improve quality of life.
4. **Anxiety and Depression**: Cannabis-based therapies are sometimes used to manage anxiety and depression, although the exact effects can vary depending on the individual and the cannabinoid profile (i.e., THC vs. CBD content).

CB2 Receptor Agonists:

1. **Inflammatory Conditions**: CB2 receptor agonists are being investigated for their role in reducing inflammation in diseases like rheumatoid arthritis, inflammatory bowel disease (IBD), and colitis. They may help reduce the severity of inflammation and improve patient outcomes.
2. **Neurodegenerative Diseases**: Because CB2 receptors have neuroprotective properties, they are being studied for their potential in treating conditions such as Alzheimer's disease, Parkinson's disease, and Huntington's disease by protecting neurons from damage caused by oxidative stress and inflammation.
3. **Pain Relief**: CB2 receptor modulators can be used to alleviate chronic pain, particularly in inflammatory and autoimmune conditions, by reducing inflammatory mediators.

4. **Cancer Therapy**: Some research suggests that CB2 activation may have anti-cancer effects by modulating immune responses and inhibiting tumor growth, though further clinical research is needed.

5. Contraindications

While cannabinoids have therapeutic potential, their use is not suitable for everyone, and there are several contraindications to consider:

1. **Psychiatric Disorders**: Cannabinoids, especially those that act on CB1 receptors (e.g., THC), may exacerbate symptoms of anxiety, depression, or psychosis in individuals with a predisposition to mental health conditions, including schizophrenia. Caution should be taken when using cannabis in these populations.
2. **Pregnancy and Lactation**: Cannabis use during pregnancy, particularly products containing THC, is generally contraindicated due to potential risks to fetal development, including low birth weight, developmental delays, and cognitive issues. THC is also excreted in breast milk and could affect infant development.
3. **Liver and Kidney Disease**: Cannabinoids are metabolized in the liver, so individuals with liver dysfunction may require dose adjustments. Likewise, caution is needed when using cannabinoids in patients with kidney disease due to potential alterations in metabolism and excretion.
4. **Drug Interactions**: Cannabinoids may interact with certain medications, such as anticoagulants (e.g., warfarin) and sedatives, altering their effects. Patients on medications that affect the liver's cytochrome P450 enzyme system should use cannabinoids with caution.
5. **History of Substance Abuse**: People with a history of substance abuse or addiction, particularly to cannabis or other psychoactive substances, should avoid using cannabinoids due to the potential for misuse or dependency.

Summary

Cannabinoid receptors (CB1 and CB2) play a crucial role in various physiological processes, such as pain modulation, appetite regulation, immune response, and inflammation. CB1 receptor activation is primarily responsible for the psychoactive effects of cannabis, whereas CB2 receptors are involved in immune modulation and inflammation.

Cannabinoid receptor modulators, including THC and CBD, have therapeutic potential for conditions like pain, nausea, appetite loss, inflammation, and neurodegenerative diseases. However, their use is contraindicated in individuals with certain psychiatric conditions, pregnant women, and those with liver or kidney dysfunction, among others.

CHAPTER 13

CHEMERIN RECEPTORS

Chemerin receptors, also known as **ChemR23** (also called **CMKLR1**), are a class of G-protein-coupled receptors (GPCRs) that are activated by the protein chemerin, a chemokine-like protein. Chemerin plays an important role in regulating immune system functions, inflammation, and metabolic processes. It acts as an endogenous ligand for the Chemerin receptor, binding to and activating the receptor to trigger various cellular responses. The Chemerin receptor is found in various tissues, including immune cells, adipose tissue, and endothelial cells.

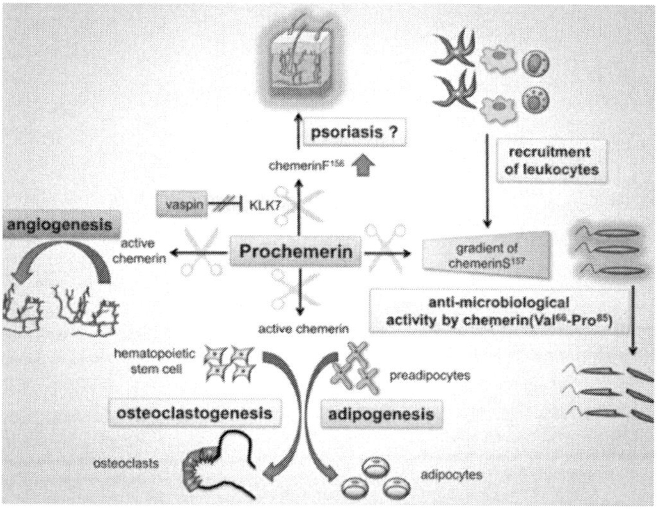

Fig. 13.1 Chemerin receptors and pharmacological actions in human body.

2. Classification of Chemerin Receptors

The primary chemerin receptor is classified as a G-protein-coupled receptor (GPCR). It has been identified as ChemR23 or CMKLR1, which stands for Chemotactic Receptor 23 or Chemerin Chemokine-Like Receptor 1. This receptor is involved in several physiological processes through its interaction with its ligand, chemerin. There are no widely recognized subtypes of the Chemerin receptor, as it primarily refers to the ChemR23 receptor.

3. Pharmacological Actions of Chemerin Receptors

The activation of chemerin receptors leads to various pharmacological effects related to inflammation, immune response, and metabolic regulation. When chemerin binds to **ChemR23**, it triggers multiple signaling pathways, such as those involving phospholipase C, calcium mobilization, and MAP kinase cascades.

Immune System Regulation and Inflammation:

1. **Chemotaxis**: One of the key actions of chemerin receptor activation is the recruitment and migration of immune cells. Chemerin promotes the chemotaxis (movement) of various immune cells, such as dendritic cells, monocytes, and T cells, to sites of inflammation or injury. This makes the receptor an important mediator in immune response and inflammatory processes.
2. **Monocyte and Dendritic Cell Activation**: Chemerin also plays a role in the activation of dendritic cells and monocytes. These cells, which are key players in the immune system, are attracted to areas of inflammation through chemerin receptor signaling.
3. **Regulation of Inflammatory Cytokine Release**: The activation of the chemerin receptor can modulate the production and release of pro-inflammatory cytokines, such as TNF-α and IL-6, by immune cells. This suggests that chemerin receptor activation can both exacerbate and modulate inflammatory responses depending on the context.

Metabolic Regulation:

1. **Adipocyte Differentiation and Function**: Chemerin has been shown to influence the differentiation of adipocytes (fat cells). It can regulate fat storage and adipose tissue function, which ties it to metabolic processes such as lipid metabolism and insulin sensitivity.
2. **Obesity and Insulin Resistance**: Chemerin levels are often elevated in obese individuals, and there is evidence suggesting that

chemerin receptor activation may contribute to the development of insulin resistance. Chemerin could be involved in the inflammatory processes associated with metabolic syndrome.

3. **Atherosclerosis**: Chemerin has been implicated in the pathogenesis of atherosclerosis, with its effects on inflammation and the recruitment of immune cells contributing to the development of arterial plaque and narrowing of blood vessels.

Neuroinflammation:

- **Central Nervous System (CNS)**: Recent research suggests that chemerin and its receptor may also be involved in neuroinflammation and the progression of neurodegenerative diseases. This could include roles in diseases such as Alzheimer's and Parkinson's, where inflammation of the CNS is a key factor in disease progression.

Angiogenesis and Vascular Remodeling:

- **Endothelial Cell Function**: The chemerin receptor is expressed on endothelial cells, which line the blood vessels. When activated, ChemR23 can influence endothelial cell behavior, including promoting angiogenesis (formation of new blood vessels) and vascular remodeling. This is important for wound healing and tissue repair.

4. Indications for Use

Research into chemerin receptor modulators is still in the early stages, but there is significant interest in the therapeutic potential of targeting the chemerin-ChemR23 axis in various disease conditions, especially those involving inflammation, metabolic disorders, and immune dysregulation.

Potential Therapeutic Applications:

1. **Anti-inflammatory Treatment**: Due to its role in immune cell recruitment and cytokine production, chemerin receptor antagonists or inhibitors could be used to treat inflammatory conditions like rheumatoid arthritis, inflammatory bowel disease, asthma, and psoriasis.
2. **Metabolic Syndrome and Obesity**: Modulation of chemerin receptor activity could have therapeutic potential in the

management of obesity and insulin resistance, particularly as chemerin levels are elevated in these conditions and contribute to inflammation and metabolic dysfunction.

3. **Cardiovascular Diseases**: Given its involvement in atherosclerosis and vascular remodeling, targeting the chemerin receptor may offer therapeutic benefits in the treatment of atherosclerosis, coronary artery disease, and other cardiovascular diseases where inflammation plays a role in the progression of the disease.
4. **Neurodegenerative Diseases**: Due to chemerin's involvement in neuroinflammation, there is the potential for chemerin receptor modulators to be developed as treatments for diseases like Alzheimer's disease and Parkinson's disease, which are characterized by inflammation in the central nervous system.
5. **Wound Healing**: Since chemerin can influence angiogenesis and vascular remodeling, it may have applications in improving wound healing and tissue repair, particularly in cases of chronic wounds or post-surgical recovery.

5. Contraindications

Given that the understanding of chemerin receptor modulation is still evolving, the contraindications are not yet fully established, but certain considerations should be taken into account:

1. **Immune System Disorders**: Inhibiting or modulating the chemerin receptor could potentially affect the immune system, particularly by reducing the recruitment of immune cells to sites of infection or injury. Therefore, chemerin receptor antagonists should be used cautiously in individuals with immunodeficiency or autoimmune disorders.
2. **Pregnancy and Lactation**: As with most novel therapies, the effects of chemerin receptor modulation during pregnancy and lactation have not been extensively studied. Therefore, its use in pregnant or breastfeeding women should be avoided unless absolutely necessary and under strict medical supervision.
3. **Cardiovascular Diseases**: While there is potential for chemerin receptor modulation to treat cardiovascular diseases, there may also be risks involved in manipulating immune cell activity and vascular remodeling. In patients with severe cardiovascular conditions, such as uncontrolled hypertension or heart failure, careful monitoring would be necessary.

4. **Metabolic Conditions**: In individuals with metabolic conditions like type 2 diabetes or **obesity**, chemerin receptor modulation may influence insulin sensitivity and fat storage, potentially leading to undesired effects. Close monitoring would be required to assess the impact on metabolic control.

Summary

Chemerin receptors (ChemR23) are involved in several physiological processes, primarily related to immune response, inflammation, and metabolic regulation. They play critical roles in recruiting immune cells to sites of inflammation, modulating adipocyte differentiation, and influencing vascular remodeling. Potential therapeutic applications include treatments for inflammatory diseases, metabolic disorders such as obesity and insulin resistance, cardiovascular diseases, and neurodegenerative conditions. However, as research progresses, the full spectrum of contraindications, risks, and benefits will become clearer, and caution is advised when targeting this receptor in certain populations.

CHAPTER 14

CHEMOKINE RECEPTORS

Chemokine receptors are a class of G-protein-coupled receptors (GPCRs) that bind to chemokines, a type of cytokine involved in immune cell recruitment and signaling. Chemokines are small proteins that mediate immune responses by directing the movement of immune cells to sites of infection, injury, or inflammation. The chemokine receptors are essential for the regulation of immune system function, inflammation, and tissue homeostasis. They play key roles in processes such as immune cell trafficking, wound healing, tissue development, and the progression of various diseases, including cancer, autoimmune disorders, and infections.

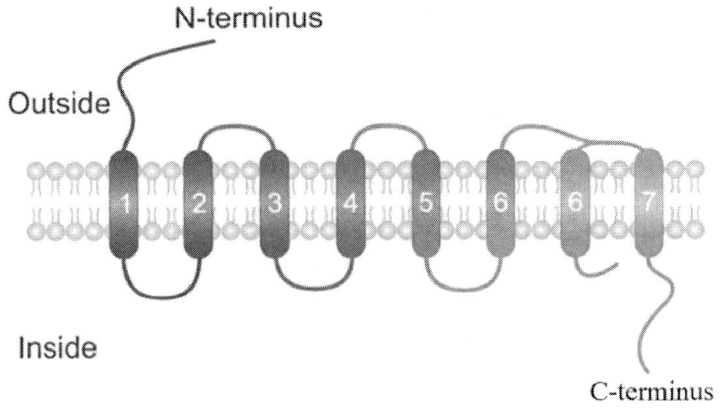

Fig 14.1 Structure of Chemokine Receptors

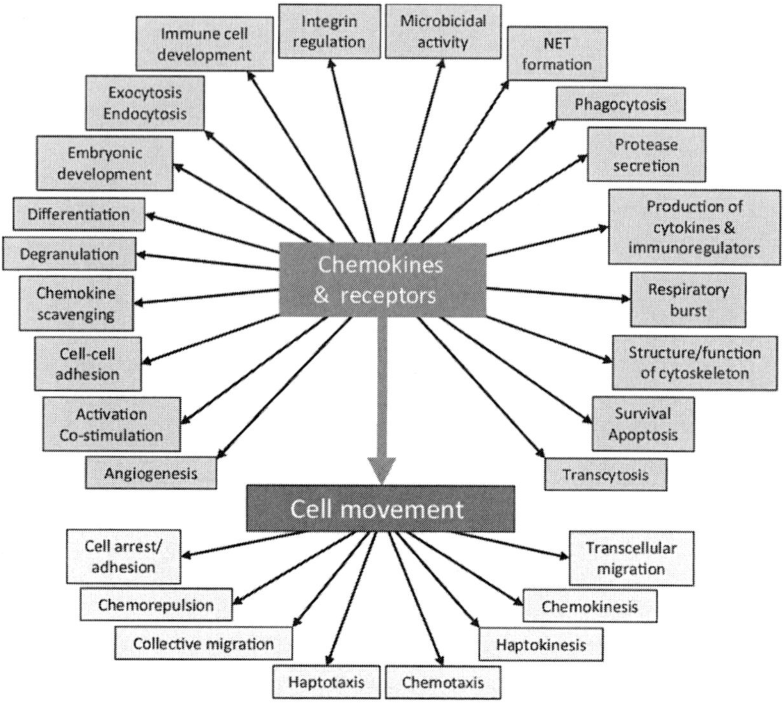

Fig. 14.2 Chemokine Receptors and actions.

Chemokine receptors are divided into two main groups based on the structure of the chemokine ligand and the receptor's biological activity:

- **CC receptors** (e.g., CCR1, CCR2, CCR3)
- **CXC receptors** (e.g., CXCR1, CXCR2, CXCR3)

These receptors typically transmit signals that influence the migration of leukocytes, angiogenesis, and inflammation.

2. Classification of Chemokine Receptors

Chemokine receptors are classified into two broad families based on the structure of the ligands that bind to them:

A. CC Chemokine Receptors (CCR):

- **Ligands**: Bind to CC chemokines, which have two adjacent cysteine residues near the N-terminus.
- **Key Receptors**:
  - **CCR1**: Involved in the migration of monocytes and dendritic cells.
  - **CCR2**: Plays a role in recruiting monocytes to sites of inflammation, particularly in diseases like atherosclerosis and arthritis.
  - **CCR3**: Involved in the recruitment of eosinophils and is important in allergic reactions and asthma.
  - **CCR4**: Involved in recruiting T cells to sites of inflammation, and plays a role in allergic responses.
  - **CCR5**: Important in the migration of T cells and monocytes, and is known for being the co-receptor used by the HIV virus to enter cells.

B. CXC Chemokine Receptors (CXCR):

1. **Ligands**: Bind to CXC chemokines, which contain an amino acid sequence with a single amino acid between the two cysteine residues.
2. **Key Receptors**:
   - ❖ **CXCR1**: Binds interleukin-8 (IL-8) and plays a role in neutrophil chemotaxis.
   - ❖ **CXCR2**: Also binds IL-8 and other related chemokines, involved in neutrophil recruitment during inflammation.
   - ❖ **CXCR3**: Associated with Th1-type immune responses and involved in the recruitment of T cells to sites of inflammation.
   - ❖ **CXCR4**: Plays a key role in hematopoiesis, development, and HIV infection, as it is a co-receptor for the HIV virus.
   - ❖ **CXCR5**: Involved in the trafficking of B cells to lymphoid follicles.

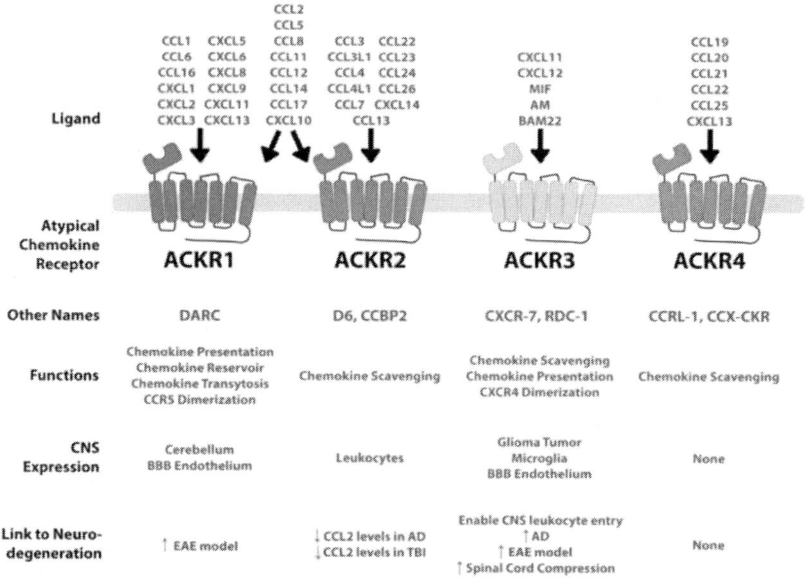

Fig. 14.3 Chemokine Receptors ligands, location and functions.

C. Other Chemokine Receptors:

- **CX3CR1**: The receptor for fractalkine, which plays a role in monocyte and microglial cell migration, and is important in neuroinflammation and atherosclerosis.

Chemokine receptors also include some non-classical receptors that are involved in specific immune responses, such as **XCR1**, which mediates the migration of dendritic cells in the lymphoid tissues.

3. Pharmacological Actions of Chemokine Receptors

Chemokine receptors mediate diverse pharmacological effects depending on the receptor type and the immune cells they regulate. The pharmacological actions of chemokine receptors primarily involve immune cell migration and the regulation of inflammation, but they also impact other physiological processes.

CC Chemokine Receptors (e.g., CCR1, CCR2, CCR5)

- **Immune Cell Migration**: Chemokine receptor activation, particularly in CCR1, CCR2, and CCR5, leads to the recruitment of monocytes, dendritic cells, T cells, and neutrophils to sites of inflammation, infection, and injury.
- **Inflammation**: These receptors contribute to the initiation and persistence of inflammation, especially in conditions like rheumatoid arthritis, atherosclerosis, and inflammatory bowel disease.
- **Role in HIV**: CCR5 is known as a coreceptor for HIV entry into host cells, and blocking CCR5 is a strategy used in the treatment of HIV.
- **Angiogenesis**: Some CC chemokine receptors are involved in the formation of new blood vessels (angiogenesis), which is crucial for tissue repair, wound healing, and tumor growth.

CXC Chemokine Receptors (e.g., CXCR1, CXCR2, CXCR4) functions

- **Neutrophil Recruitment**: CXCR1 and CXCR2 are involved in the recruitment of neutrophils to areas of infection or injury, contributing to acute inflammation and tissue repair.
- **Hematopoiesis**: CXCR4 plays a key role in the development and movement of hematopoietic cells (stem cells, progenitor cells) within the bone marrow.
- **Cancer Metastasis**: CXCR4 is implicated in the metastatic spread of cancer cells, particularly in breast cancer, lymphoma, and other malignancies. The receptor supports cancer cell migration to distant organs.
- **Angiogenesis and Tissue Repair**: Some CXC receptors, such as CXCR4, are involved in angiogenesis, which helps repair blood vessels and tissues following injury.

Other Chemokine Receptors

- **Fractalkine (CX3CR1)**: Plays a critical role in the migration of monocytes and microglial cells, especially in neuroinflammatory conditions, such as in neurodegenerative diseases like Alzheimer's disease.

- **CXCR5**: Regulates B cell migration and plays a role in immune responses by guiding B cells to germinal centers in secondary lymphoid organs.

4. Indications for Use

Chemokine receptors are targeted for therapeutic purposes in a range of conditions where immune system regulation, inflammation, and cell migration are key processes. Potential indications include:

1. **Inflammatory Diseases**: In conditions such as rheumatoid arthritis, inflammatory bowel disease, asthma, and psoriasis, blocking specific chemokine receptors can reduce the recruitment of inflammatory cells and alleviate symptoms.
2. **HIV/AIDS**: CCR5 antagonists, such as maraviroc, are used in the treatment of HIV infection by blocking the receptor that HIV uses to enter host cells, thereby preventing viral replication.
3. **Cancer**: Chemokine receptor antagonists, especially those targeting CXCR4, are being investigated as potential therapies for cancer metastasis by preventing the migration of cancer cells to secondary sites.
4. **Neurological Diseases**: Targeting CX3CR1 and other chemokine receptors may provide therapeutic benefits in neurodegenerative diseases like Alzheimer's and Parkinson's disease, as these receptors play a role in microglial activation and neuroinflammation.
5. **Wound Healing and Tissue Repair**: Modulating chemokine receptor activity can help improve tissue repair and wound healing, particularly in the context of chronic wounds or post-surgical recovery.

5. Contraindications

While chemokine receptor modulators hold potential in treating a variety of conditions, they also come with risks and contraindications:

1. **Immunosuppressive Effects**: Blocking chemokine receptors can impair immune cell migration and function, leading to an increased risk of infection. Therefore, inhibitors of chemokine receptors should be used cautiously in individuals with immunodeficiency or in those who are at high risk of infections.

2. **Cancer**: Although chemokine receptor blockers have the potential to prevent cancer metastasis, they could also interfere with the immune system's ability to fight tumors. Caution should be taken in cancer patients, especially when targeting receptors like **CXCR4**.
3. **Cardiovascular Diseases**: Some chemokine receptors, particularly CCR2 and CXCR4, are involved in vascular remodeling and angiogenesis. Inhibiting these receptors could affect tissue repair and blood vessel formation, potentially complicating conditions like heart disease or stroke.
4. **Pregnancy**: The effects of chemokine receptor inhibitors on fetal development are not fully understood, so their use should be avoided during **pregnancy** unless the potential benefit justifies the risk.
5. **Neurological Disorders**: In patients with neuroinflammatory diseases, such as **multiple sclerosis**, the modulation of chemokine receptors might alter neuroimmune interactions and potentially worsen disease progression. Use in such conditions should be approached with caution.

Summary

Chemokine receptors are integral to immune system regulation, inflammation, and cell migration. By mediating the movement of immune cells to sites of infection, injury, and inflammation, chemokine receptors play critical roles in the immune response and tissue homeostasis. Pharmacologically, these receptors have therapeutic potential in a range of diseases, including inflammatory conditions, HIV, cancer, and neurological diseases. However, careful consideration must be given to the potential risks, such as immune suppression, cancer metastasis, and cardiovascular complications, when using chemokine receptor modulators as treatment options.

CHAPTER 15

CHOLECYSTOKININ RECEPTORS

Cholecystokinin (CCK) receptors are a group of G-protein-coupled receptors (GPCRs) that mediate the biological actions of cholecystokinin, a peptide hormone found in the gastrointestinal (GI) tract and brain. CCK plays a pivotal role in regulating various digestive processes, including the stimulation of gallbladder contraction and pancreatic enzyme secretion, as well as influencing satiety and digestion. CCK receptors are present throughout the body, with the primary receptors being CCK1 and CCK2.

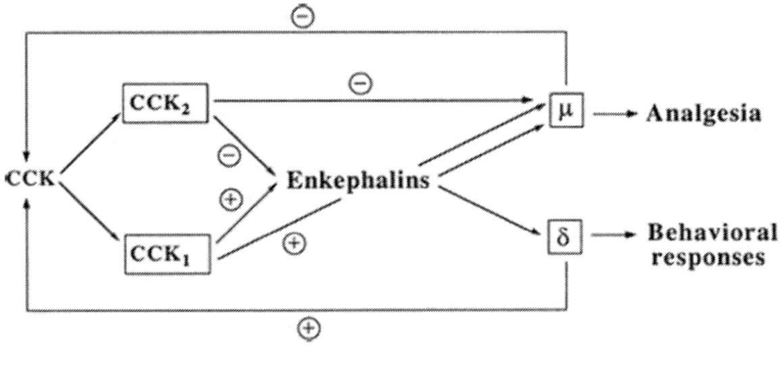

Fig. 15.1 Role of CCK receptors and pharmacological actions.

2. Classification of Cholecystokinin Receptors

There are two main types of cholecystokinin receptors based on their binding affinity and physiological roles:

A. CCK1 Receptor (CCK-A Receptor)

- **Location**: Primarily located in the pancreas, gallbladder, stomach, and the central nervous system (CNS).
- **Function**: CCK1 receptors are involved in regulating gallbladder contraction, pancreatic enzyme secretion, gastric acid secretion,

and satiety. In the CNS, they influence feeding behavior and appetite.
- **Ligand**: CCK-8 (octapeptide form of cholecystokinin) is the primary endogenous ligand, although the receptor can also bind longer forms of CCK.

B. CCK2 Receptor (CCK-B Receptor)

- **Location**: Primarily located in the CNS (especially in the brainstem), and also in the gastrointestinal tract, particularly in the stomach and pancreas.
- **Function**: The CCK2 receptor is involved in regulating gastric acid secretion, gastric motility, and some central processes such as anxiety and pain perception. It is also the receptor for gastrin, another gastrointestinal peptide hormone, which has overlapping actions with CCK.
- **Ligand**: CCK and gastrin both bind to CCK2 receptors, with gastrin being the natural ligand in some tissues.

3. Pharmacological Actions of Cholecystokinin Receptors

Cholecystokinin receptors mediate a variety of physiological effects depending on the receptor subtype and location of action.

CCK1 Receptor (CCK-A) Pharmacological Actions

1. **Gallbladder Contraction**: One of the primary roles of CCK1 receptor activation is the contraction of the gallbladder, which aids in the release of bile into the duodenum for the digestion of fats.
2. **Pancreatic Enzyme Secretion**: CCK1 receptor activation stimulates the secretion of digestive enzymes from the pancreas, particularly amylase, lipase, and proteases. This enhances the breakdown of carbohydrates, fats, and proteins in the small intestine.
3. **Gastric Acid Secretion**: CCK1 receptors also play a role in the secretion of gastric acid from the stomach, which aids in digestion.
4. **Satiety and Appetite Regulation**: CCK is known to promote feelings of fullness (satiety) by acting on the central nervous system. When released after food intake, it signals the brain to reduce hunger, contributing to appetite control. This action is mediated by CCK1 receptors in the brain, particularly in areas involved in feeding behavior such as the hypothalamus.

5. **Gastric Motility**: CCK1 receptor activation also slows gastric emptying, allowing for more efficient digestion of nutrients.

CCK2 Receptor (CCK-B) Pharmacological Actions

1. **Gastric Acid Secretion**: Similar to CCK1 receptors, CCK2 receptors are involved in the stimulation of gastric acid secretion in the stomach, promoting digestion.
2. **Gastric Motility**: CCK2 receptors play a role in regulating gastric motility, facilitating proper food transit through the stomach and intestines.
3. **Central Nervous System Effects**: The CCK2 receptor is implicated in various central effects, such as modulation of anxiety and stress responses. Activation of CCK2 receptors in the brainstem and other brain regions can influence mood, arousal, and anxiety.
4. **Pain Perception**: CCK2 receptors have been linked to the modulation of pain, with receptor activation potentially enhancing pain sensitivity or promoting pain relief, depending on the context.

4. Indications for Use

Cholecystokinin receptor agonists and antagonists are explored for therapeutic use in several medical conditions:

CCK1 Receptor (CCK-A) Agonists and Antagonists

1. **Gallstone Disease**: CCK1 receptor agonists may help in the treatment of gallstones by promoting gallbladder contraction and enhancing bile secretion, although this approach is still being investigated.
2. **Digestive Disorders**: Agents that target the CCK1 receptor can be used to treat conditions related to inadequate pancreatic enzyme secretion, such as pancreatic insufficiency and chronic pancreatitis, by stimulating enzyme release from the pancreas.
3. **Obesity and Weight Management**: Since CCK1 activation promotes satiety, CCK receptor agonists are being studied for their potential in weight loss and the management of obesity. However, the use of CCK agonists for this purpose requires careful regulation due to possible side effects such as nausea.
4. **Postprandial Satiety**: CCK1 receptor agonists could help in the treatment of conditions involving impaired satiety signaling, such

as in obesity and prader-willi syndrome, by promoting early feelings of fullness during meals.

CCK2 Receptor (CCK-B) Agonists and Antagonists Actions

1. **Gastric Acid Secretion Disorders**: CCK2 receptor antagonists could be used in conditions involving excessive gastric acid secretion, such as gastritis, peptic ulcers, or Zollinger-Ellison syndrome, to reduce gastric acid production.
2. **Anxiety and Stress Disorders**: CCK2 receptor antagonists or inverse agonists are being investigated for their potential to reduce anxiety and stress responses, as activation of the CCK2 receptor in the brain is associated with anxiety-like behavior.
3. **Pain Management**: CCK2 receptor antagonists are being explored as potential analgesics, as CCK2 receptor activation has been implicated in pain sensitivity and modulation.
4. **Cancer**: CCK2 receptor antagonists may be useful in reducing gastric acid secretion associated with certain types of gastric cancer or in modulating the growth and metastasis of certain tumors, although more research is needed.

5. Contraindications

The use of cholecystokinin receptor agonists and antagonists must be considered carefully due to potential contraindications and side effects, including:

- **Gallbladder Disease**: Since CCK1 receptor agonists induce gallbladder contraction, they should be used cautiously in patients with gallstones or gallbladder disease, as this may exacerbate symptoms or lead to gallstone migration and obstruction.
- **Pancreatic Conditions**: In individuals with pancreatitis or severe pancreatic insufficiency, the use of CCK1 receptor agonists could worsen symptoms by overstimulating pancreatic enzyme secretion.
- **Peptic Ulcer Disease**: CCK2 receptor agonists can increase gastric acid secretion and may worsen symptoms of peptic ulcers or gastritis. These should be avoided in patients with active ulcers.
- **Anxiety and Mood Disorders**: Given the involvement of CCK2 receptors in anxiety and stress responses, antagonists should be used cautiously in patients with mood disorders, as blocking these receptors could interfere with normal emotional regulation.

- **Pregnancy**: As with many pharmacological agents, the use of CCK receptor modulators in pregnancy should be avoided unless the potential benefit outweighs the risk. The effects of CCK agonists and antagonists on fetal development are not well-established.
- **Gastrointestinal Obstruction**: In cases of intestinal obstruction or conditions causing abnormal gastrointestinal motility, CCK agonists may exacerbate symptoms by altering motility and gastric emptying.

Summary

Cholecystokinin receptors (CCK1 and CCK2) are critical regulators of digestive processes, including gallbladder contraction, pancreatic enzyme secretion, and gastric acid production. They also play significant roles in appetite regulation, satiety, and central processes like anxiety and pain. Pharmacological agents targeting these receptors have therapeutic potential in managing conditions such as obesity, pancreatic insufficiency, gastritis, anxiety, and pain disorders. However, careful consideration of contraindications and potential side effects, particularly in individuals with gallbladder disease, peptic ulcers, or pancreatic conditions, is essential when using CCK receptor modulators in clinical practice.

CHAPTER 16

CLASS FRIZZLED G PROTEIN-COUPLED RECEPTORS (FRIZZLED GPCRS)

Frizzled receptors (FZDs) constitute a subfamily of Class F G protein-coupled receptors (GPCRs). They function as the primary receptors for Wnt proteins, which are secreted glycoproteins involved in intercellular signaling pathways that govern embryonic development, tissue homeostasis, and cellular processes such as proliferation, differentiation, and migration. The term "Frizzled" originates from phenotypic abnormalities observed in Drosophila mutants, manifesting in disoriented cuticular bristles due to disrupted Wnt signaling (Logan &Nusse, 2004).

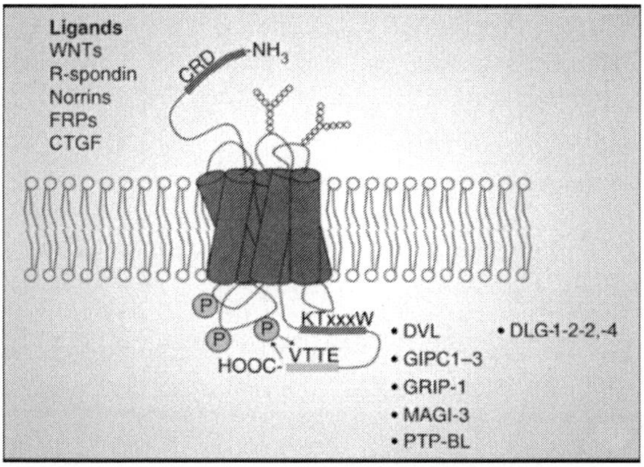

Fig. 16.1 Structure of Frizzled receptors (FZDs)

2. Classification

The Frizzled family comprises ten distinct receptors (FZD1 to FZD10) in humans, each with a conserved N-terminal cysteine-rich domain (CRD) for Wnt binding. They are classified under Class F GPCRs, along with the

Smoothened (SMO) receptor, which is structurally similar but functions in the Hedgehog signaling pathway (Katritch et al., 2013).

- **FZD1–FZD10**: Mediators of Wnt signaling
- **SMO (Smoothened)**: Involved in Hedgehog signaling, often studied alongside FZDs due to structural similarities

3. **Pharmacological Actions** Frizzled GPCRs are integral to the Wnt signaling cascade, which can be broadly categorized into:
4. **Canonical Wnt/β-catenin Pathway**: Activation leads to accumulation and nuclear translocation of β-catenin, driving transcription of Wnt target genes involved in proliferation and survival (Clevers&Nusse, 2012).

- **Non-Canonical Pathways**:
    - *Planar Cell Polarity (PCP) Pathway*: Regulates cytoskeletal dynamics and cell polarity (Veeman et al., 2003).
    - *Wnt/Ca2+ Pathway*: Modulates intracellular calcium levels, activating downstream effectors like protein kinase C (PKC) and calcium/calmodulin-dependent protein kinase II (CAMKII) (Kuhl et al., 2000).

Frizzled receptors interact with Dishevelled (Dvl) proteins, G proteins, and β-arrestins, transmitting signals that influence embryogenesis, tissue regeneration, and oncogenesis (Schulte & Bryja, 2007).

4. Indications

Pharmacological targeting of Frizzled GPCRs is under investigation in various pathological conditions:

- **Cancer**: Overactivation of Wnt/FZD signaling is implicated in colorectal, breast, liver, and pancreatic cancers (Anastas & Moon, 2013).
- **Fibrotic Disorders**: Pulmonary, hepatic, and renal fibrosis (Henderson et al., 2010).
- **Bone Metabolic Diseases**: Osteoporosis and other disorders of bone density and formation (Baron & Kneissel, 2013).
- **Neurodegenerative Diseases**: Potential neuroprotective roles in Alzheimer's and Parkinson's disease (Inestrosa& Varela-Nallar, 2014).
- **Wound Healing and Regenerative Medicine**: Enhancing tissue repair via Wnt/FZD activation (Whyte et al., 2012).

- **Ophthalmologic Conditions**: Retinal vascular development and diabetic retinopathy (Lobov et al., 2005).

5. Contraindications

While clinical application is still emerging, potential contraindications include:

- **Pregnancy**: Wnt signaling is essential during embryogenesis; its inhibition may result in developmental anomalies (MacDonald et al., 2009).
- **Immunological Disorders**: Monoclonal antibodies or Wnt inhibitors may trigger immune responses.
- **Gastrointestinal and Hematopoietic Disorders**: Wnt signaling maintains intestinal epithelium and hematopoietic stem cells; disruption could impair normal physiology (Luis et al., 2012).
- **Chronic Suppression Risks**: Long-term inhibition might impair tissue regeneration and stem cell function.

References

1. Anastas, J. N., & Moon, R. T. (2013). WNT signalling pathways as therapeutic targets in cancer. *Nature Reviews Cancer*, 13(1), 11–26.
2. Baron, R., &Kneissel, M. (2013). WNT signaling in bone homeostasis and disease: from human mutations to treatments. *Nature Medicine*, 19(2), 179–192.
3. Clevers, H., &Nusse, R. (2012). Wnt/β-catenin signaling and disease. *Cell*, 149(6), 1192–1205.
4. Henderson, W. R. et al. (2010). Wnt/β-catenin pathway: a target for asthma and other diseases. *Therapeutic Advances in Respiratory Disease*, 4(3), 151–166.
5. Inestrosa, N. C., & Varela-Nallar, L. (2014). Wnt signaling in the nervous system and in Alzheimer's disease. *Journal of Molecular Cell Biology*, 6(1), 64–74.
6. Katritch, V., Cherezov, V., & Stevens, R. C. (2013). Structure-function of the G protein–coupled receptor superfamily. *Annual Review of Pharmacology and Toxicology*, 53, 531–556.
7. Kuhl, M. et al. (2000). Wnt/Ca2+ signaling: a novel branch of the Wnt pathway. *Cell*, 100(5), 591–602.

8. Lobov, I. B. et al. (2005). Wnt signaling mediates angiogenic responses and vascular development in the retina. *Nature Neuroscience*, 8(5), 541–548.
9. Logan, C. Y., &Nusse, R. (2004). The Wnt signaling pathway in development and disease. *Annual Review of Cell and Developmental Biology*, 20, 781–810.
10. Luis, T. C. et al. (2012). Wnt signaling strength regulates normal hematopoiesis and its deregulation is involved in leukemia development. *Leukemia*, 26(3), 414–421.
11. MacDonald, B. T., Tamai, K., & He, X. (2009). Wnt/β-catenin signaling: components, mechanisms, and diseases. *Developmental Cell*, 17(1), 9–26.
12. Schulte, G., & Bryja, V. (2007). The Frizzled family of unconventional G-protein-coupled receptors. *Trends in Pharmacological Sciences*, 28(10), 518–525.
13. Veeman, M. T. et al. (2003). Zebrafish prickle, a modulator of noncanonical Wnt/Fz signaling, regulates gastrulation movements. *Current Biology*, 13(8), 680–685.
14. Whyte, J. L. et al. (2012). Wnt signaling and injury repair. *Cold Spring Harbor Perspectives in Biology*, 4(5), a008078.

CHAPTER 17

COMPLEMENT PEPTIDE RECEPTORS

Complement peptide receptors are a class of G protein-coupled receptors (GPCRs) that specifically bind to activated cleavage products of the complement system, particularly the anaphylatoxins C3a and C5a. These receptors play crucial roles in modulating immune responses, mediating inflammation, and coordinating host defense mechanisms. They are predominantly expressed on immune cells, including neutrophils, monocytes, eosinophils, and mast cells.

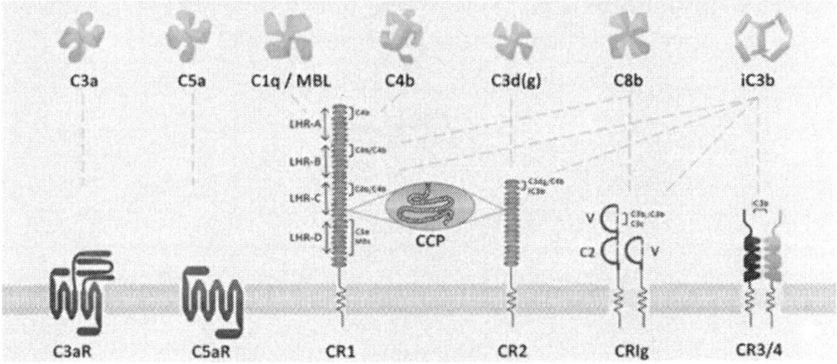

Fig 17. 1 Structure of Complement Peptide Receptors.

2. Classification

The main complement peptide receptors include:

1. **C3a Receptor (C3aR)**: Binds to the C3a anaphylatoxin. Involved in chemotaxis, cytokine release, and degranulation.
2. **C5a Receptor 1 (C5aR1/CD88)**: A classical GPCR that binds to C5a, triggering robust pro-inflammatory responses.

3. **C5a Receptor 2 (C5aR2/C5L2/GPR77)**: An atypical receptor that binds C5a and its des-Arg form; modulates or antagonizes C5aR1 signaling and may function as a decoy receptor.

3. Pharmacological Actions

Upon activation, complement peptide receptors trigger downstream signaling cascades through G-protein-mediated and β-arrestin-dependent pathways:

1. **Pro-inflammatory effects**: Including vasodilation, chemotaxis, reactive oxygen species (ROS) generation, and release of inflammatory mediators.
2. **Immune cell recruitment**: Essential for host defense and pathogen clearance.
3. **C5aR1 antagonism**: Can reduce excessive inflammation and tissue injury.
4. **C5aR2 modulation**: May exert anti-inflammatory or immune-regulatory effects, depending on context.

4. Indications

Therapeutic targeting of complement receptors is under clinical and preclinical investigation for several disorders:

- **Sepsis and systemic inflammatory response syndrome (SIRS)**
- **Autoimmune diseases**: Rheumatoid arthritis, systemic lupus erythematosus
- **Ischemia-reperfusion injury**: In myocardial infarction, stroke, or transplantation
- **Neurological diseases**: Alzheimer's disease, multiple sclerosis
- **Chronic inflammatory and allergic conditions**: Asthma, chronic obstructive pulmonary disease

5. Contraindications

Although therapeutic inhibitors are promising, potential contraindications may include:

- **Risk of infections**: Due to impaired innate immune responses
- **Pregnancy**: Complement system plays a role in fetal development; modulation may be unsafe
- **Immunocompromised patients**: Suppression of complement activity may exacerbate vulnerability
- **Pre-existing autoimmune dysregulation**: Unintended immune suppression or dysregulation

References

1. Klos, A., Tenner, A. J., Johswich, K. O., Ager, R. R., Reis, E. S., & Köhl, J. (2009). The role of the anaphylatoxins in health and disease. *Molecular Immunology*, 46(14), 2753–2766.
2. Guo, R. F., & Ward, P. A. (2005). Role of C5a in inflammatory responses. *Annual Review of Immunology*, 23, 821–852.
3. Monk, P. N., Scola, A. M., Madala, P., & Fairlie, D. P. (2007). Function, structure and therapeutic potential of complement C5a receptors. *British Journal of Pharmacology*, 152(4), 429–448.
4. Bamberg, C. E., Mackay, C. R., Lee, H., Zahra, D., Jackson, J., Lim, Y. S., ... & Housley, G. D. (2010). The C5a receptor (C5aR2) modulates C5aR1-mediated responses. *Nature*, 465(7296), 108–112.
5. Ricklin, D., Reis, E. S., &Lambris, J. D. (2016). Complement in disease: a defence system turning offensive. *Nature Reviews Nephrology*, 12(7), 383–401.

CHAPTER 18

CORTICOTROPIN-RELEASING RECEPTORS (CRH RECEPTORS)

1. Introduction

Corticotropin-releasing hormone (CRH) receptors are pivotal components of the neuroendocrine system that modulate the body's response to stress. These receptors belong to the class B family of G protein-coupled receptors (GPCRs) and are primarily activated by CRH and related peptides such as urocortins. Through their activation, CRH receptors regulate the hypothalamic-pituitary-adrenal (HPA) axis and influence a wide range of physiological processes including mood, anxiety, immune responses, cardiovascular regulation, and gastrointestinal motility.

2. Definition

CRH receptors are transmembrane proteins that bind corticotropin-releasing hormone and urocortins, initiating a cascade of intracellular signaling events. These receptors play an essential role in integrating endocrine, autonomic, and behavioral responses to stress. They are primarily expressed in the brain and peripheral tissues and are involved in mediating the physiological adaptations required during both acute and chronic stress conditions.

3. Classification

CRH receptors are divided into two major subtypes based on their genetic and functional properties:

- **CRH Receptor 1 (CRHR1)**: this receptor localized mainly in the pituitary gland, cerebral cortex, hippocampus, cerebellum, and amygdala.
    - It Has a high affinity for CRH and Urocortin 1 (Ucn1).

  - It Plays a central role in initiating the HPA axis response by stimulating the release of adrenocorticotropic hormone (ACTH) from the anterior pituitary.
- **CRH Receptor 2 (CRHR2)**:
  - It Found in peripheral tissues such as the heart, gastrointestinal tract, and skin, as well as in certain brain regions like the hypothalamus and lateral septum.
  - It Preferentially binds Urocortins 2 and 3.
  - It Modulates cardiovascular and gastrointestinal responses and is involved in stress-coping mechanisms.

Each receptor subtype is encoded by a distinct gene and may exist in multiple isoforms due to alternative splicing, which can affect receptor localization and function.

4. Pharmacological Actions

CRH receptors are primarily coupled to the Gs protein, which activates adenylate cyclase and increases intracellular cyclic adenosine monophosphate (cAMP) levels. This activation leads to a variety of downstream effects:

1. **CRHR1 Functions**:
   - ❖ **Endocrine response**: Stimulates ACTH secretion, leading to cortisol production by the adrenal cortex.
   - ❖ **Behavioral effects**: Involved in anxiety, fear, and arousal responses.
   - ❖ **Immunomodulation**: Alters cytokine profiles and immune cell trafficking.
   - ❖ **Neurotransmission**: Affects dopaminergic, serotonergic, and noradrenergic systems.
2. **CRHR2 Functions**:
   - ❖ **Cardiovascular modulation**: Enhances vasodilation and cardiac output, providing a compensatory mechanism during stress.
   - ❖ **Gastrointestinal regulation**: Modulates motility and secretion in the GI tract.
   - ❖ **Emotional regulation**: Plays a role in adaptive stress responses and anxiolysis.

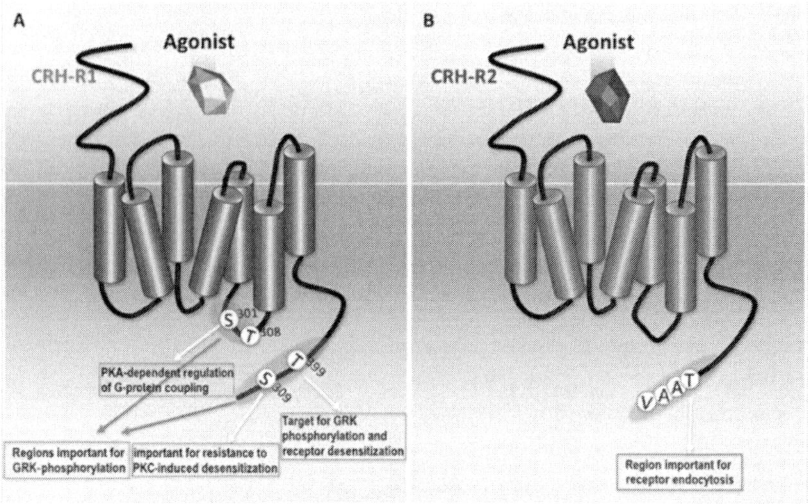

Fig 18.1 Corticotropin-releasing hormone (CRH) receptors types and actions.

5. Therapeutic Indications:

Targeting CRH receptors offers promising therapeutic potential for a variety of disorders characterized by dysregulated stress responses:

- **Psychiatric Disorders**:
  - Major depressive disorder (MDD)
  - Generalized anxiety disorder (GAD)
  - Post-traumatic stress disorder (PTSD)
- **Gastrointestinal Disorders**:
  - Irritable bowel syndrome (IBS)
  - Inflammatory bowel disease (IBD)
- **Endocrine Disorders**:
  - Cushing's disease (CRH overproduction or ectopic ACTH syndrome)
- **Cardiovascular Conditions**:
  - Heart failure and stress-induced cardiomyopathy
- **Inflammatory and Autoimmune Diseases**:
  - Rheumatoid arthritis and systemic lupus erythematosus

CRH receptor antagonists, particularly selective CRHR1 blockers, are under clinical investigation for these conditions.

6. Contraindications and Precautions

Despite their therapeutic promise, the pharmacological modulation of CRH receptors must be approached cautiously due to the complexity of their physiological roles:

- **Pregnancy and Lactation**: CRH plays a role in placental function and timing of labor. Antagonism may interfere with normal gestation and fetal development.
- **Adrenal Insufficiency**: In patients with adrenal suppression or insufficiency, further downregulation of the HPA axis can be hazardous.
- **Infectious Diseases**: Immunosuppressiveeffec

References

1. Spiess, J., Rivier, J., Rivier, C., & Vale, W. (1981). Primary structure of corticotropin-releasing factor from ovine hypothalamus. *Proceedings of the National Academy of Sciences*, 78(10), 6517–6521.
2. Bale, T. L., & Vale, W. W. (2004). CRF and CRF receptors: Role in stress responsivity and other behaviors. *Annual Review of Pharmacology and Toxicology*, 44, 525–557.
3. Heinrichs, S. C., & Koob, G. F. (2004). Corticotropin-releasing factor in brain: A role in activation, arousal, and affect regulation. *Journal of Pharmacology and Experimental Therapeutics*, 311(2), 427–440.
4. Zorrilla, E. P., Tache, Y., & Koob, G. F. (2003). Nibbling at CRF receptor control of gastrointestinal function and emotion. *Current Opinion in Pharmacology*, 3(6), 614–619.
5. Kehne, J. H. (2007). CRF receptor antagonists as potential antidepressants. *Current Opinion in Investigational Drugs*, 8(1), 12–20.

CHAPTER 19

DOPAMINE

1. Introduction

Dopamine, a catecholaminergic neurotransmitter, is central to a wide spectrum of neurobiological functions ranging from motor activity and endocrine regulation to cognition and emotional processing. Its actions are mediated via five distinct dopamine receptor subtypes, which belong to the G protein-coupled receptor (GPCR) superfamily. The dopaminergic system is distributed throughout the central nervous system (CNS) and plays a vital role in both physiological and pathological processes, making it a key target for pharmacological interventions in neuropsychiatric and neurodegenerative disorders.

2. Definition of Dopamine Receptors

Dopamine receptors are membrane-spanning proteins that transduce extracellular dopamine signals into intracellular responses via activation of heterotrimeric G proteins. Upon binding dopamine, these receptors modulate intracellular signaling pathways including cyclic adenosine monophosphate (cAMP), phospholipase C, and mitogen-activated protein kinase (MAPK) cascades. They are predominantly located in the brain regions associated with reward, motivation, motor control, and endocrine regulation such as the striatum, prefrontal cortex, hypothalamus, and pituitary gland.

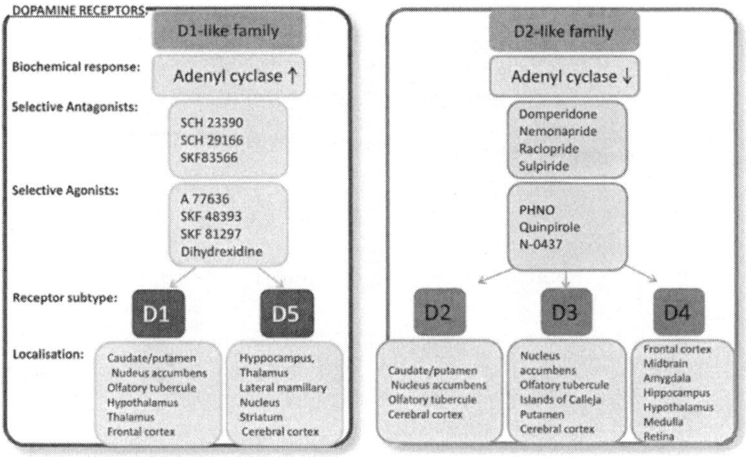

Fig. 19.1 Dopamine receptors subtypes and classification, functions.

3. Classification of Dopamine Receptors

Dopamine receptors are divided into two families based on their structural and functional characteristics:

I. **D1-like Receptors**
   - ❖ Includes D1 and D5 receptor subtypes.
   - ❖ Coupled to Gs proteins that stimulate adenylate cyclase, resulting in increased cAMP production.
   - ❖ Typically mediate excitatory effects on neurons.

II. **D2-like Receptors**
   - ❖ Includes D2, D3, and D4 receptor subtypes.
   - ❖ Coupled to Gi/o proteins that inhibit adenylate cyclase and reduce intracellular cAMP.
   - ❖ Predominantly exert inhibitory effects.

Each receptor subtype has a distinct anatomical distribution, ligand affinity, and functional profile. For instance, D1 receptors are most abundant in the striatum and prefrontal cortex, while D2 receptors are found both pre- and post-synaptically in several regions including the basal ganglia and limbic system.

4. Pharmacological Actions

The physiological effects of dopamine are mediated through the activation or inhibition of downstream effectors upon receptor binding:

I. **D1 Receptors**
- It Stimulate neuronal excitability and synaptic plasticity.
- It Enhances cognitive performance, particularly working memory and attention.
- It Potentiate the effects of glutamatergic transmission.

II. **D2 Receptors**
- It Act as autoreceptors to inhibit dopamine release.
- It Decrease neuronal firing and modulate behavioral responses.
- It Primary target of most antipsychotic agents.

III. **D3 and D4 Receptors**
- It Involved in modulation of emotional and cognitive functions.
- It Play a role in reinforcement and addiction behaviors.

IV. **D5 Receptors**
- It Regulate synaptic plasticity and are implicated in emotional reactivity.

Pharmacologically, dopamine receptors are the target of a range of agonists, antagonists, and partial agonists used in the treatment of CNS disorders.

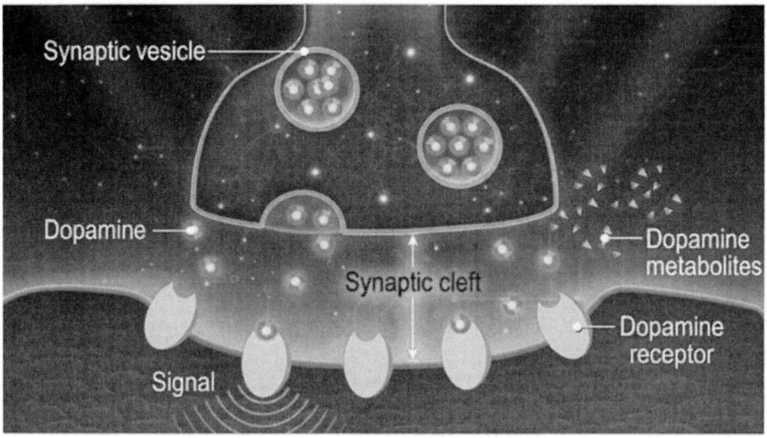

Fig 19.2 Release of Dopamine and binding with receptors.

5. Therapeutic Indications

Dopamine receptor modulators are clinically employed in several medical conditions:

I. **Parkinson's Disease**: Dopamine agonists (e.g., pramipexole, ropinirole) target D2-like receptors to compensate for dopaminergic deficit.
II. **Schizophrenia and Psychotic Disorders**: Antipsychotics (e.g., haloperidol, risperidone) primarily block D2 receptors to reduce positive symptoms.
III. **Bipolar Disorder**: Mood stabilizers with D2 antagonistic effects help manage manic episodes.
IV. **Prolactinomas and Hyperprolactinemia**: D2 agonists (e.g., bromocriptine, cabergoline) suppress prolactin secretion.
V. **Attention Deficit Hyperactivity Disorder (ADHD)**: Stimulants (e.g., methylphenidate) enhance dopaminergic tone by inhibiting reuptake.
VI. **Restless Legs Syndrome (RLS)**: Dopaminergic agents are often first-line treatments.

6. Contraindications and Precautions

Although beneficial, dopamine-targeting agents must be used with caution under certain conditions:

I. **Psychosis**: Dopamine agonists may exacerbate psychotic symptoms.
II. **Cardiovascular Disease**: Agents like dopamine and dopaminergic agonists can cause arrhythmias, hypotension, or hypertension.
III. **Pregnancy and Lactation**: Dopaminergic agents may interfere with hormonal balance and fetal development.
IV. **Substance Use Disorders**: Dopaminergic stimulation has high abuse potential.
V. **Renal or Hepatic Impairment**: May require dosage adjustments due to altered metabolism and excretion.

Summary

Dopamine receptors are crucial in maintaining the delicate balance of neuronal activity underlying motor control, cognition, emotion, and endocrine function. The ability to pharmacologically modulate these receptors has revolutionized the management of numerous CNS disorders. Future research aimed at receptor subtype specificity and biased signaling may unlock more precise and efficacious therapeutic options with fewer adverse effects.

Clinical Importance

Dopamine D_2 receptor — Antipsychotic-induced parkinsonism (drug-induced extrapyramidal symptoms)

Vignette idea: Older adult starts haloperidol for psychosis then develops bradykinesia and rigidity; discuss D_2 antagonism in nigrostriatal pathway, differential diagnosis (Parkinson disease vs DIP), and management.

Reference: Feldman M, et al. Updated Perspectives on Management of Drug-Induced Parkinsonism. *Clin Neuropharmacol/Review.* 2022.

References

1. Beaulieu, J. M., &Gainetdinov, R. R. (2011). The physiology, signaling, and pharmacology of dopamine receptors. *Pharmacological Reviews*, 63(1), 182–217.
2. Missale, C., Nash, S. R., Robinson, S. W., Jaber, M., & Caron, M. G. (1998). Dopamine receptors: From structure to function. *Physiological Reviews*, 78(1), 189–225.
3. Sibley, D. R. (1999). New insights into dopaminergic receptor function using antisense and genetically altered animals. *Annual Review of Pharmacology and Toxicology*, 39(1), 313–341.
4. Seeman, P. (2006). Targeting the dopamine D2 receptor in schizophrenia. *Expert Opinion on Therapeutic Targets*, 10(4), 515–531.
5. Volkow, N. D., & Morales, M. (2015). The brain on drugs: From reward to addiction. *Cell*, 162(4), 712–725

CHAPTER 20

ESTROGEN RECEPTORS (ERS)

Estrogen Receptors (ERs) are a family of intracellular nuclear receptors that mediate the actions of endogenous estrogen hormones, such as E2 (17\beta-estradiol). As members of the nuclear receptor superfamily, their primary function is to act as ligand-activated transcription factors, regulating gene expression throughout the body.

I. Classification and Structure

There are two major subtypes of estrogen receptors, each encoded by a different gene and exhibiting distinct tissue distributions and binding affinities for ligands:

Receptor Subtype	**Gene**	**Primary Location & Function**
Estrogen Receptor Alpha (ER\alpha)	ESR1	Predominant in breast, uterus, hypothalamus, and liver. Often associated with cell proliferation and growth.
Estrogen Receptor Beta (ER\beta)	ESR2	Predominant in ovaries, prostate, lung, bone, and CNS. Often associated with differentiation, regulation, and anti-proliferative effects.

Both ER\alpha and ER\beta share a common structural organization typical of nuclear receptors, possessing six functional domains (A-F). The most pharmacologically relevant domains are:

- **DNA-Binding Domain** (DBD, **Domain C):** Contains two zinc-finger motifs that bind to specific DNA sequences called Estrogen Response Elements (EREs).

- **Ligand-Binding Domain** (LBD, **Domain E**)**:** The pocket where estrogen or pharmacological ligands bind. This domain also mediates dimerization and binding to co-regulatory proteins.

II. Mechanism of Action

ERs mediate their effects through two primary mechanisms:

1. Genomic Pathway (Classical Mechanism)

This is the slower mechanism, resulting in changes in protein synthesis and cellular function.

- **Binding:** E2 diffuses across the cell membrane and binds to an inactive, cytoplasmic ER (either ER\alpha or ER\beta).
- **Activation:** Ligand binding causes the receptor to undergo a conformational change, leading to homodimerization (ER\alpha/ ER\alpha or ER\beta/ER\beta) or heterodimerization (ER\alpha/ ER\beta).
- **Transcription:** The activated dimer translocates to the nucleus and binds to EREs in the promoter region of target genes. The receptor recruits either co-activator or co-repressor proteins, which modify chromatin structure and either initiate or suppress transcription.

2. Non-Genomic Pathway (Rapid Mechanism)

This is a faster process occurring within seconds to minutes, independent of gene transcription. A small pool of ERs is tethered to the plasma membrane (often via palmitoylation). Upon ligand binding, these membrane ERs quickly activate intracellular signaling cascades, such as the MAPK and PI3K pathways, affecting ion channel activity or other fast cellular processes.

III. Pharmacological Ligands and Modulators

The primary goal of ER pharmacology is to selectively activate or inhibit receptor function in specific tissues to treat disease while minimizing adverse effects.

Table 20.1 clical use of Agonist and antagonist of ERs.

Drug Class	Mechanism	Example Agents	Clinical Use
Agonists	Bind to and activate ERs in all tissues.	17\beta-Estradiol, Conjugated Estrogens	Hormone Replacement Therapy (HRT) for menopausal symptoms; prevention of osteoporosis.
Antagonists (SERDs)	**Selective Estrogen Receptor Degraders.** Bind to ERs and destabilize them, leading to their proteasomal degradation.	**Fulvestrant**	Treatment of hormone receptor-positive breast cancer; effective against Tamoxifen-resistant tumors.
SERMs	**Selective Estrogen Receptor Modulators.** Act as **agonists** in some tissues (e.g., bone) and **antagonists** in others (e.g., breast/endometrium).	**Tamoxifen, Raloxifene**	**Tamoxifen:** Breast cancer treatment (antagonist in breast, partial agonist in endometrium). **Raloxifene:** Osteoporosis prevention (agonist in bone, antagonist in breast/uterus).
Aromatase Inhibitors	Block the enzyme Aromatase, which synthesizes estrogen from androgens, thereby lowering circulating estrogen levels.	Anastrozole, Letrozole	Used for postmenopausal ER positive breast cancer, where peripheral estrogen synthesis is the primary source.

IV. Clinical and Pathophysiological Relevance

ER function is implicated in multiple physiological and pathological processes:

- **Breast Cancer:** Approximately 75\% of breast cancers are ER-positive (ER+). Targeting the ER is the cornerstone of treatment using SERMs (like Tamoxifen) and SERDs (like Fulvestrant) to block proliferative signaling.
- **Osteoporosis:** Estrogen prevents bone resorption. SERMs like Raloxifene selectively act as ER agonists in bone to preserve bone density without stimulating breast or uterine tissue.
- **Cardiovascular System:** Estrogen has complex cardiovascular effects. ER\beta activation is often associated with protective effects (vasodilation, anti-inflammatory), while ER\alpha may mediate proliferative effects.
- **Reproductive System:** ERs are essential for uterine and ovarian function, controlling the menstrual cycle.

The future of ER pharmacology lies in developing highly selective ligands (known as SERMs or SERDs) that can specifically target ER\alpha or ER\beta in a tissue-selective manner to maximize therapeutic benefits while avoiding side effects like endometrial hyperplasia (caused by Tamoxifen's agonist activity in the uterus).

CHAPTER 21

ENDOTHELIN RECEPTORS

1. Introduction

Endothelin receptors are critical regulators of vascular tone, cellular proliferation, and hormone production. They are G protein-coupled receptors (GPCRs) that mediate the biological effects of endothelins (ETs)—a family of potent vasoconstrictive peptides. The endothelin system, including endothelin-1 (ET-1), endothelin-2 (ET-2), and endothelin-3 (ET-3), is involved in various physiological processes and is implicated in several pathological conditions such as hypertension, pulmonary arterial hypertension (PAH), heart failure, and cancer.

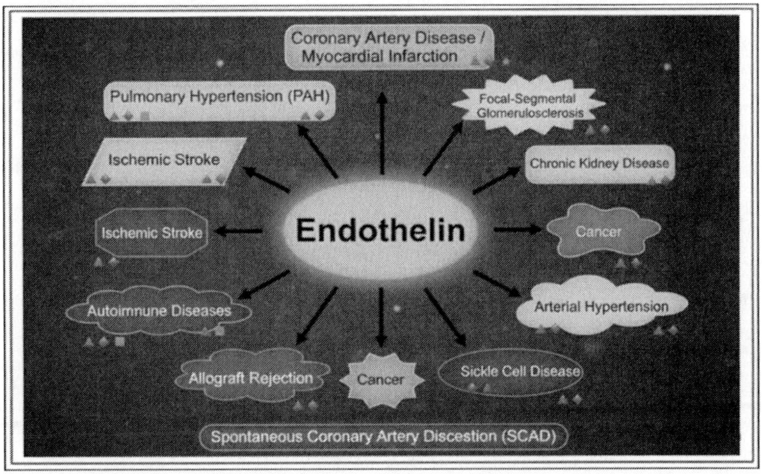

Fig 21.1 Endothelin receptors and pharmacological actions.

2. Definition

Endothelin receptors are membrane-bound GPCRs that bind endothelins with high affinity and transduce their signals via activation of intracellular pathways. The most studied isoform, ET-1, acts predominantly through two receptor subtypes: ETA and ETB.

3. Classification of Endothelin Receptors

There are two primary receptor subtypes:

A. **ETA Receptor**:
   - High affinity for ET-1 and ET-2.
   - Coupled to Gq and G11 proteins, leading to activation of phospholipase C (PLC), resulting in intracellular calcium mobilization.
   - Located primarily on vascular smooth muscle cells, mediating **vasoconstriction** and cell proliferation.

B. **ETB Receptor**:
   - Binds all three endothelins (ET-1, ET-2, ET-3) with equal affinity.
   - Found on endothelial cells (ETB1 subtype) and vascular smooth muscle cells (ETB2 subtype).
   - ETB1 mediates vasodilationvia nitric oxide (NO) and prostacyclin release.
   - ETB2 can contribute to vasoconstriction under certain conditions.

4. Pharmacological Actions

Endothelin receptor activation leads to diverse physiological and pathological effects:

I. **ETA Receptor Activation**:
   - Vasoconstriction
   - Vascular smooth muscle proliferation
   - Inflammation
   - Fibrosis
   - Cardiac hypertrophy

II. **ETB Receptor Activation**:
   - Endothelial-dependent vasodilation
   - Clearance of ET-1 from circulation

- ❖ Inhibition of cell proliferation
- ❖ Promotion of natriuresis (renal ETB)

Intracellular signaling pathways involve:

- ❖ PLC/IP3/DAG/Ca^{2+} pathway
- ❖ Rho kinase (ROCK)
- ❖ MAPK and ERK1/2 cascades
- ❖ NADPH oxidase-mediated ROS production

5. Indications

Endothelin receptor antagonists (ERAs) are used or investigated in various conditions:

- **Pulmonary Arterial Hypertension (PAH)**: Bosentan, ambrisentan, and macitentan (ET receptor antagonists) reduce pulmonary vascular resistance and improve exercise capacity.
- **Systemic Hypertension and Heart Failure**: Investigational; ERAs may reduce afterload and fibrosis.
- **Chronic Kidney Disease**: Due to antifibrotic and antiproteinuric effects.
- **Raynaud's Phenomenon and Scleroderma**: ERAs like bosentan prevent digital ulcers.
- **Cancer**: Overexpression of ET-1 and ETA contributes to tumor proliferation and angiogenesis; targeted therapies are under evaluation.

6. Contraindications and Precautions

While ERAs provide therapeutic benefits, their use may be contraindicated or require caution in the following conditions:

- **Hepatic Impairment**: Bosentan is hepatotoxic; liver enzyme monitoring is essential.
- **Pregnancy**: Teratogenic potential; contraindicated in pregnancy.
- **Anemia**: ERAs can decrease hemoglobin levels.
- **Hypotension**: Due to vasodilatory effects, caution is advised in patients with low blood pressure.
- **Concomitant use with cyclosporine or glyburide**: Risk of elevated plasma concentrations and liver toxicity.

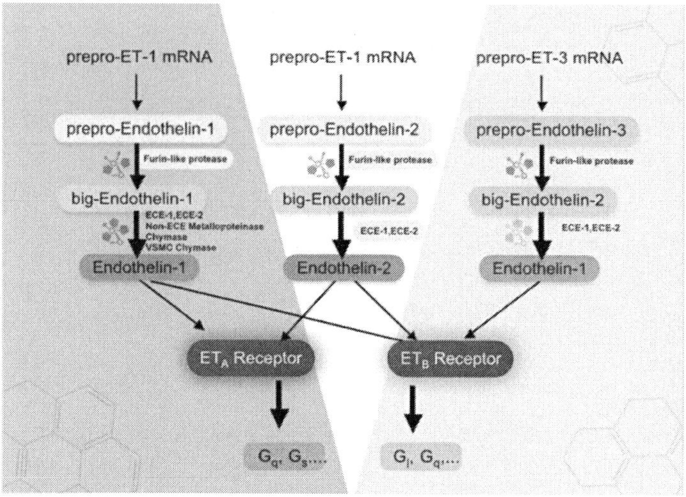

Fig. 21.2 Endothelin receptors and its types.

Figure: In red, components of the pre-proET-1 -> ECE-1 -> ET-1 ->ET_A receptor axis are shown which is responsible for the development of embryonic cephalic and cardiac neural crest-derived craniofacial and cardiac outflow structures, vasoconstriction, cell growth, and inflammation, among other actions. In blue, the components of the preproET-3 ->ECE-1 ->ET-3 ->ET_B receptor axis are shown which is important for the development of neural crest-derived epidermal melanocytes and enteric neurons, natriuresis, and melanocyte growth.

7. Summary

Endothelin receptors play a dual role in vascular homeostasis, with ETA and ETB subtypes mediating opposing effects. The development of selective and dual ERAs has revolutionized the management of PAH and holds promise for other diseases. Future research aims to refine receptor selectivity and minimize adverse effects for broader clinical application.

References

1. Davenport, A. P., Hyndman, K. A., Dhaun, N., et al. (2016). Endothelin. *Pharmacological Reviews*, 68(2), 357–418. https://doi.org/10.1124/pr.115.011833

2. Galiè, N., Manes, A., Negro, L., Palazzini, M., Bacchi-Reggiani, M. L., &Branzi, A. (2009). A meta-analysis of randomized controlled trials in pulmonary arterial hypertension. *European Heart Journal*, 30(4), 394–403.
3. Kohan, D. E., Barton, M. (2014). Endothelin and endothelin antagonists in chronic kidney disease. *Kidney International*, 86(5), 896–904.
4. Kedzierski, R. M., & Yanagisawa, M. (2001). Endothelin system: the double-edged sword in health and disease. *Annual Review of Pharmacology and Toxicology*, 41(1), 851–876.
5. Iglarz, M., &Clozel, M. (2010). At the heart of tissue: endothelin system and end-organ damage. *Clinical Science*, 119(10), 453–463.

CHAPTER 22

SEROTONIN (5-HYDROXYTRYPTAMINE OR 5-HT) RECEPTOR

1. Introduction

Serotonin (5-hydroxytryptamine or 5-HT) is a biogenic monoamine involved in diverse physiological functions including mood regulation, sleep, appetite, cognition, and vascular tone. The effects of serotonin are mediated through a complex family of serotonin receptors, collectively known as 5-HT receptors. These receptors are distributed extensively in the central and peripheral nervous systems and are vital therapeutic targets in neuropsychiatric, gastrointestinal, and cardiovascular disorders.

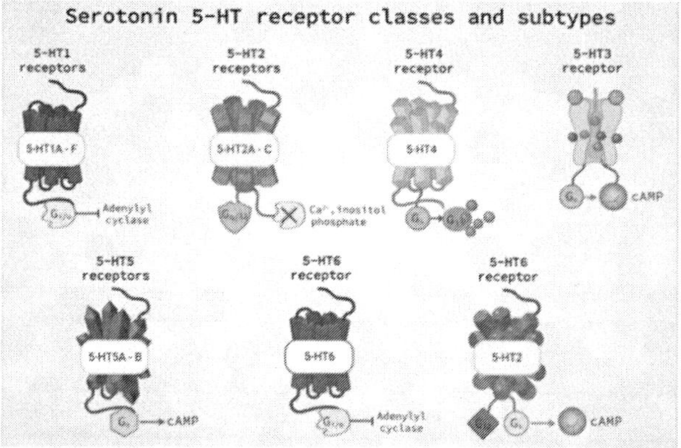

Fig. 22.1 Serotonin (5-hydroxytryptamine or 5-HT) Receptor and sub types.

2. Definition

5-HT receptors are a family of structurally and functionally distinct membrane proteins that respond to serotonin binding by initiating intracellular signaling cascades. Most 5-HT receptors are G protein-coupled receptors (GPCRs), except for the 5-HT3 subtype, which is a ligand-gated ion channel. Their activation modulates neuronal excitability, neurotransmitter release, and hormonal secretion.

3. Classification of 5-HT Receptors

The 5-HT receptor family is divided into seven major classes (5-HT1 to 5-HT7), with further subtypes within some classes:

I. **5-HT1 Receptors** (GPCRs coupled to Gi/o)
   - Subtypes: 5-HT1A, 1B, 1D, 1E, 1F
   - Function: Inhibition of adenylate cyclase, reducing cAMP; often inhibitory

II. **5-HT2 Receptors** (GPCRs coupled to Gq/11)
   - Subtypes: 5-HT2A, 2B, 2C
   - Function: Activation of phospholipase C; generally excitatory

III. **5-HT3 Receptors** (Ligand-gated ion channels)
   - Function: Cation-selective ion channel causing rapid depolarization

IV. **5-HT4, 5-HT6, 5-HT7 Receptors** (GPCRs coupled to Gs)
   - Function: Stimulation of adenylate cyclase; excitatory effects

V. **5-HT5 Receptors** (Poorly understood)
   - Subtypes: 5-HT5A (functional), 5-HT5B (non-functional in humans)
   - Function: Presumed inhibitory

4. Pharmacological Actions

The physiological effects of 5-HT receptor activation vary by subtype and tissue localization:

- **5-HT1A:** Anxiolytic, antidepressant effects; auto-inhibition in raphe nuclei
- **5-HT1B/1D:** Cranial vasoconstriction; target for anti-migraine drugs
- **5-HT2A:** CNS excitation, hallucinations, platelet aggregation
- **5-HT2C:** Appetite suppression, mood regulation
- **5-HT3:** Emesis control, gut motility; involved in nausea and pain perception
- **5-HT4:** Gastrointestinal prokinetic effects
- **5-HT6/7:** Cognitive enhancement, circadian rhythm regulation

Table 22.1 list of 5-HT receptor subtypes and therie location and function.

Subtype	Signal transduction	Localization	Function	Selective Agonist	Selective Antagonist
5-HT_1A	Inhibition of AC	Hippocampus	Autoreceptor	8-OA-DPAT	WAY 100135
5-HT_1B	Inhibition of AC	Substantia nigra	Autoreceptor	-	-
5-HT_1D	Inhibition of AC	Cranial blood vessels	Vasoconstriction	Sumatriptan	-
5-HT_1E	Inhibition of AC	Cortex	-	-	-
5-HT_1F	Inhibition of AC	Brain, Periphery	-	-	-
5-HT_2A	Activation of PLC	Platelet, smooth muscle, cerebral cortex	Platelet aggre^n,Contra^n, Neuronal excitation	DOI	Ketanserin, Resperidone
5-HT_2B (D-receptor)	Activation of PLC	Stomach fundus	Contraction	DOI	LY53857
5-HT_2C	Activation of PLC	Choroid plexus	-	DOI	LY53857, Mesulergine
5-HT_3 (M-receptor)	Ion channel	PNS	Neuronal excitat^n	2-methyl-5HT	Ondansetron, Tropisetron
5-HT_4	Activation of AC	GI tract, Hippocampus	Neuronal excitat^n	Renzapride	GR113808
5-HT_5A	Inhibition of AC	Hippocampus	Unknown	-	-
5-HT_5B	Unknown	Unknown	Unknown	-	-
5-HT_6	Activation of AC	Striatum	Unknown	-	-
5-HT_7	Activation of AC	Hypothalamus, Intestine	Unknown	-	-

5. Therapeutic Indications

- **Depression and Anxiety:** SSRIs and SNRIs increase synaptic 5-HT; 5-HT1A partial agonists (e.g., buspirone)
- **Migraine:** 5-HT1B/1D agonists (e.g., sumatriptan)
- **Schizophrenia and Psychosis:** 5-HT2A antagonists (e.g., atypical antipsychotics)
- **Nausea and Vomiting:** 5-HT3 antagonists (e.g., ondansetron)
- **IBS and GI disorders:** 5-HT4 agonists (e.g., prucalopride)
- **Obesity:** 5-HT2C agonists (e.g., lorcaserin - withdrawn due to safety concerns)

6. Contraindications and Precautions

- **Serotonin Syndrome:** Risk with polypharmacy involving serotonergic agents
- **Pregnancy/Lactation:** Caution with 5-HT drugs affecting fetal development
- **Cardiac Risk:** 5-HT2B agonism is associated with valvulopathy
- **GI Obstruction:** Avoid prokinetic 5-HT4 agents in bowel obstruction
- **QT Prolongation:** Risk with some 5-HT3 antagonists (e.g., ondansetron)

Summary

Serotonin receptors represent a highly diversified and therapeutically rich receptor family. Their subtypes are intricately involved in regulating central and peripheral functions. Understanding their pharmacodynamics enables the development of targeted therapies with improved efficacy and safety profiles.

Clinical Importance

5-HT$_3$ receptor — Ondansetron and drug-induced QT prolongation / torsades de pointes (case reports)

Vignette idea: Post-operative patient receives IV ondansetron then develops syncope and is found to have torsades de pointes; discuss 5-HT$_3$ antagonism, QT-prolonging risk, and clinical safe-use limits.

Reference / Cases: Lee DY, et al. Torsades de Pointes after Ondansetron Infusion in 2 Patients. *Case reports.* 2017; plus meta-analyses on QT prolongation risk

References

1. Hoyer, D., Hannon, J. P., & Martin, G. R. (2002). Molecular, pharmacological and functional diversity of 5-HT receptors. *Pharmacology Biochemistry and Behavior*, 71(4), 533–554.
2. Barnes, N. M., & Sharp, T. (1999). A review of central 5-HT receptors and their function. *Neuropharmacology*, 38(8), 1083–1152.
3. Nichols, D. E., & Nichols, C. D. (2008). Serotonin receptors. *Chemical Reviews*, 108(5), 1614–1641.
4. Berger, M., Gray, J. A., & Roth, B. L. (2009). The expanded biology of serotonin. *Annual Review of Medicine*, 60, 355–366.
5. Meltzer, H. Y., & Massey, B. W. (2011). The role of serotonin receptors in the action of atypical antipsychotic drugs. *Current Opinion in Pharmacology*, 11(1), 59–67.

CHAPTER 23

G PROTEIN-COUPLED RECEPTORS (GPCRS)

1. Introduction

G protein-coupled receptors (GPCRs), also referred to as seven-transmembrane domain receptors, constitute the most expansive and functionally diverse group of membrane proteins in the human genome. They regulate a wide array of physiological processes including sensory perception (vision, taste, smell), neurotransmission, cardiovascular regulation, immune responses, and endocrine signaling. The structural versatility and signaling capacity of GPCRs make them a central focus in both basic biomedical research and pharmaceutical development. It is estimated that approximately 30–40% of all currently marketed drugs target GPCRs either directly or indirectly.

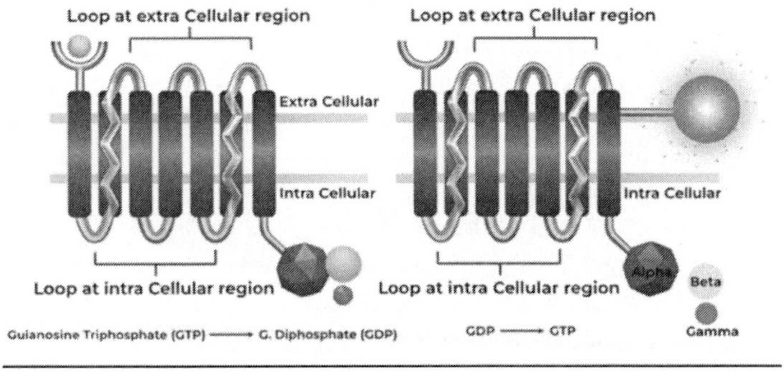

Fig. 23.1 G protein-coupled receptors structure.

2. Definition

GPCRs are defined as a superfamily of integral membrane proteins that translate extracellular stimuli into intracellular signals via activation of heterotrimeric guanine nucleotide-binding proteins (G proteins). They are characterized structurally by seven transmembrane α-helices connected by three extracellular and three intracellular loops, with an extracellular N-terminus and intracellular C-terminus. Ligand binding induces conformational changes in the receptor, facilitating the exchange of GDP for GTP on the α-subunit of the associated G protein, ultimately initiating downstream signal transduction pathways.

3. Classification of GPCRs

GPCRs can be categorized based on their sequence homology, ligand specificity, and signaling mechanisms. The most widely accepted classification system is the GRAFS system, which comprises five major families:

I. **G (Glutamate family)**
   - ❖ Includes metabotropic glutamate receptors and GABA-B receptors
   - ❖ Large extracellular domains; primarily Class C receptors

II. **R (Rhodopsin family)**
   - ❖ The largest and most studied class
   - ❖ Includes adrenergic, dopamine, serotonin, and opioid receptors

III. **A (Adhesion family)**
   - ❖ Contains long N-terminal domains involved in cell-cell interactions
   - ❖ Often implicated in immune regulation

IV. **F (Frizzled/Taste2 family)**
   - ❖ Includes Frizzled receptors involved in Wnt signaling and taste receptors

V. **S (Secretin family)**
   - ❖ Binds peptide hormones like secretin, glucagon, and vasoactive intestinal peptide (VIP)

4. Pharmacological Actions

GPCRs are activated by an extensive range of ligands, including biogenic amines (e.g., serotonin, dopamine), peptides (e.g., angiotensin II, glucagon), lipids (e.g., prostaglandins), nucleotides, and sensory stimuli. Upon activation, the associated G proteins are subdivided into four main types:

- **Gs (stimulatory)** – Activates adenylate cyclase → increases cAMP → activates protein kinase A (PKA)
- **Gi/o (inhibitory)** – Inhibits adenylate cyclase → decreases cAMP → reduces PKA activity
- **Gq/11** – Activates phospholipase C (PLC) → generates IP3 and DAG → mobilizes intracellular Ca^{2+} and activates protein kinase C (PKC)
- **G12/13** – Regulates the Rho family of GTPases → affects cell shape and motility

In addition to G protein-dependent pathways, GPCRs can initiate G protein-independent signaling via β-arrestins, which mediate receptor desensitization, internalization, and scaffolding for MAPK and other kinase pathways.

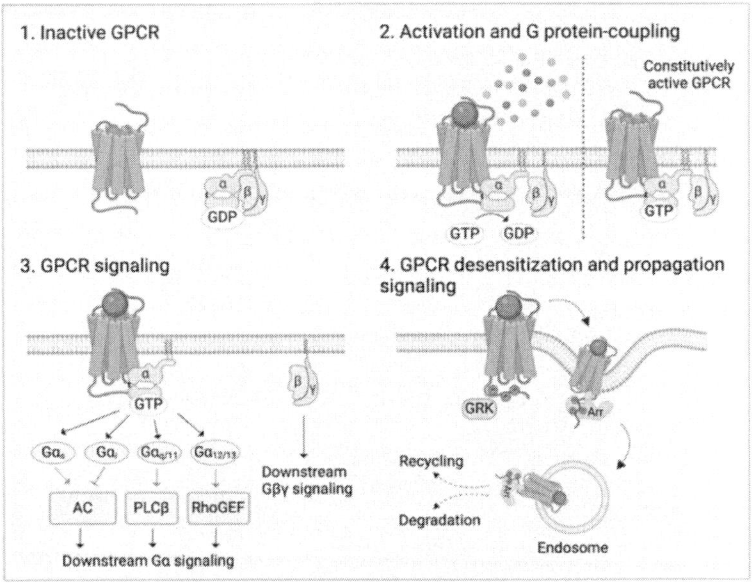

Fig. 23.2G protein-coupled receptors and their activation.

5. Therapeutic Indications

Owing to their central role in numerous physiological functions, GPCRs are implicated in the pathogenesis of various diseases and serve as prime pharmacological targets:

I. **Cardiovascular Diseases**
   - Beta-blockers (e.g., atenolol, metoprolol) for hypertension and arrhythmias
   - Angiotensin II receptor antagonists for heart failure

II. **Neurological and Psychiatric Disorders**
   - Dopamine receptor antagonists (e.g., haloperidol) for schizophrenia
   - Serotonin receptor modulators (e.g., SSRIs, buspirone) for depression and anxiety

III. **Respiratory Disorders**
   - β2-adrenergic agonists (e.g., salbutamol) for asthma and COPD

IV. **Gastrointestinal Disorders**
   - 5-HT3 receptor antagonists (e.g., ondansetron) for chemotherapy-induced nausea

V. **Endocrine and Metabolic Disorders**
   - GLP-1 receptor agonists (e.g., exenatide) for type 2 diabetes

VI. **Immunological and Oncological Conditions**
   - Chemokine receptor blockers (e.g., maraviroc) in HIV/AIDS and autoimmune conditions

6. Contraindications and Precautions

Despite their therapeutic benefits, GPCR-targeting drugs must be used cautiously due to potential adverse effects and contraindications:

A. **Pre-existing Cardiac Conditions**
   - β-agonists may induce tachyarrhythmias
   - β-blockers may worsen bradycardia or heart block

B. **Psychiatric Disorders**
   - Dopamine agonists may exacerbate psychosis
   - Serotonin modulators may cause serotonin syndrome when combined

C. **Pregnancy and Lactation**
   - Many GPCR ligands cross the placenta or are excreted in breast milk

D. **Hepatic and Renal Impairment**
   - Altered metabolism or clearance of GPCR drugs can increase toxicity

E. **Drug Interactions**
   - GPCR-targeting agents may interact with other CNS depressants or stimulants, increasing adverse effects

F. **Desensitization and Tolerance**
   - ❖ Chronic exposure to agonists can lead to receptor downregulation or tolerance

7. Summary

G protein-coupled receptors are integral to the cellular response to extracellular stimuli and play essential roles in homeostatic regulation. Their versatility and ubiquitous expression make them crucial targets for therapeutic intervention across a spectrum of disorders. Advances in structural biology, biased agonism, and allosteric modulation hold promise for developing next-generation drugs with improved specificity and reduced side effects.

Clinical Importance

Case/Study of antagonist binding kinetics at a GPCR

Citation: Ramsey SJ, Attkins NJ, Fish R, van der Graaf PH. Quantitative pharmacological analysis of antagonist binding kinetics at CRF_1 receptors in vitro and in vivo. Br J Pharmacol. 2011 Oct;164(3):992-1007. doi:10.1111/j.1476-5381.2011.01390.x.

Summary: This study explores in detail how antagonists of the ¬CRF_1 receptor bind, comparing in vitro and in vivo kinetics. It examines differences in insurmountable vs non-competitive behaviour of ligands, and links them to receptor kinetics.

Relevance: You can use this as a clinical-pharmacology-type case where receptor kinetics matter (e.g., antagonist efficacy changed by binding off-rate). Useful for chapters on "receptor kinetics" or "non-competitive vs competitive antagonism".

References

1. Pierce, K. L., Premont, R. T., & Lefkowitz, R. J. (2002). Seven-transmembrane receptors. *Nature Reviews Molecular Cell Biology*, 3(9), 639–650.

2. Hauser, A. S., Attwood, M. M., Rask-Andersen, M., Schiöth, H. B., &Gloriam, D. E. (2017). Trends in GPCR drug discovery: New agents, targets and indications. *Nature Reviews Drug Discovery*, 16(12), 829–842.
3. Insel, P. A., Tang, C. M., Hahntow, I., & Michel, M. C. (2007). Impact of GPCRs in clinical medicine: Genetic variants and drug targets. *Biochimica et Biophysica Acta (BBA) - Biomembranes*, 1768(4), 994–1005.
4. Luttrell, L. M. (2005). Composition and function of G protein-coupled receptor signalosomes. *Biochemical Journal*, 385(Pt 3), 557–564.
5. Bockaert, J., & Pin, J. P. (1999). Molecular tinkering of G protein-coupled receptors: An evolutionary success. *The EMBO Journal*, 18(7), 1723–1729.
6. Rosenbaum, D. M., Rasmussen, S. G. F., & Kobilka, B. K. (2009). The structure and function of G-protein-coupled receptors. *Nature*, 459(7245), 356–363.
7. Sriram, K., & Insel, P. A. (2018). G protein-coupled receptors as targets for approved drugs: How many targets and how many drugs? *Molecular Pharmacology*, 93(4), 251–258.

CHAPTER 24

GAMMA-AMINOBUTYRIC ACID (GABA)

1. Introduction

Gamma-Aminobutyric Acid (GABA) is the principal inhibitory neurotransmitter in the central nervous system (CNS), playing a crucial role in regulating neuronal excitability and maintaining synaptic balance. GABA exerts its effects through two main classes of receptors: ionotropic $GABA_a$ receptors and metabotropic $GABA_e$ receptors. These receptors are critical pharmacological targets for a wide range of neurological and psychiatric disorders.

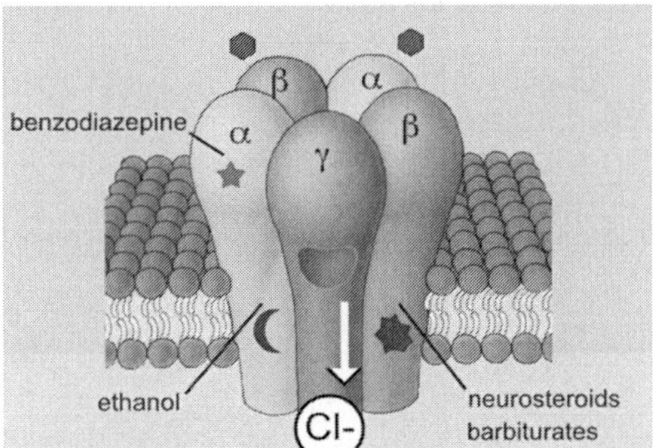

Fig. 24.1 Gamma-Aminobutyric Acid (GABA) structure.

2. Definition

GABA receptors are protein complexes located on neuronal membranes that bind GABA to mediate inhibitory neurotransmission. They are divided into:

- **GABAff receptors (GABA-A and GABA-C)**: Ligand-gated chloride ion channels

- **GABA$_e$ receptors**: G-protein-coupled receptors (GPCRs) that regulate downstream intracellular signaling pathways

3. Classification of GABA Receptors

I. **GABAff (Ionotropic)**
   - **GABA-A Receptors**: Pentameric chloride channels that mediate fast synaptic inhibition
     Subunits: α (1-6), β (1-3), γ (1-3), δ, ε, θ, π, ρ (1-3)
   - **GABA-C Receptors**: Considered a subtype of GABA-A, composed primarily of ρ subunits

II. **GABA$_e$ (Metabotropic)**
   - G-protein-coupled receptor that mediates slow and prolonged inhibitory effects
   - Primarily located in the brain and spinal cord

4. Pharmacological Actions

GABA receptor activation leads to:

- **GABA-A**: Rapid influx of Cl^- ions → Hyperpolarization of postsynaptic membrane → Inhibition of action potential firing
- **GABA-B**: Activation of G-proteins → Inhibition of adenylate cyclase → Decrease in cAMP → Modulation of ion channels (e.g., opening of K^+ channels, inhibition of Ca^{2+} channels)

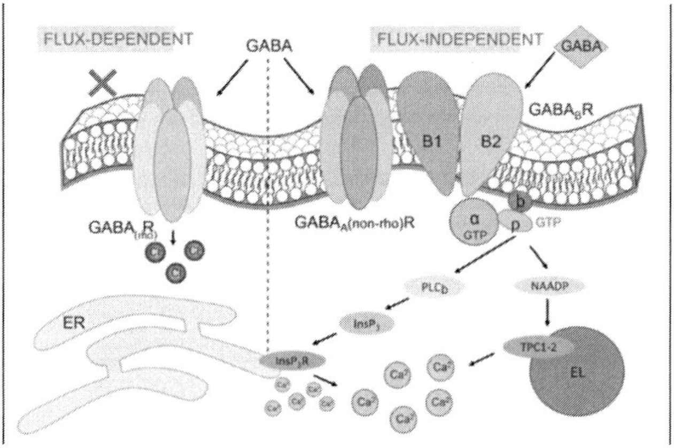

Fig. 24.2 Gamma-Aminobutyric Acid (GABA) and its mechanism of action.

5. Therapeutic Indications

A. **Anxiety Disorders**: Benzodiazepines (e.g., diazepam) enhance GABA-A receptor activity
B. **Epilepsy**: Barbiturates and vigabatrin increase GABAergic activity
C. **Muscle Spasticity**: Baclofen (GABA-B agonist)
D. **Insomnia**: Non-benzodiazepine hypnotics (e.g., zolpidem) targeting GABA-A
E. **Anesthesia**: Propofol and etomidate enhance GABA-A function

6. Contraindications and Precautions

- **Pregnancy**: Some GABAergic drugs are teratogenic (e.g., valproate)
- **Liver Disease**: Hepatic metabolism is impaired for many GABA-targeting drugs
- **Substance Abuse**: Benzodiazepines and barbiturates have high abuse potential
- **Respiratory Disorders**: CNS depressants may worsen respiratory function

Summary

GABA receptors are pivotal regulators of neuronal inhibition and are key therapeutic targets in various CNS disorders. The ongoing development of subtype-selective ligands offers promise for more precise modulation of GABAergic signaling with reduced adverse effects.

Clinical Importance

GABA_A receptor — Flumazenil reversal of benzodiazepine toxicity

Vignette idea: Elderly patient with benzodiazepine over-sedation reversed with flumazenil infusion; cover benzodiazepine binding site modulation of GABA_A, risks (seizure), and indications for use. Reference: An H, et al. Flumazenil in benzodiazepine overdose. *Br J Clin Pharmacol.* 2016 (review/case examples).

References

1. Olsen, R. W., & Sieghart, W. (2009). GABA A receptors: Subtypes provide diversity of function and pharmacology. *Neuropharmacology*, 56(1), 141–148.
2. Bowery, N. G., & Enna, S. J. (2000). Gamma-aminobutyric acid B receptors: First of the functional metabotropic heterodimers. *Journal of Pharmacology and Experimental Therapeutics*, 292(1), 2–7.
3. Rudolph, U., &Knoflach, F. (2011). Beyond classical benzodiazepines: Novel therapeutic potential of GABA A receptor subtypes. *Nature Reviews Drug Discovery*, 10(9), 685–697.
4. Bettler, B., & Tiao, J. Y. (2006). Molecular diversity, trafficking and subcellular localization of GABA B receptors. *Pharmacology & Therapeutics*, 110(3), 533–543.
5. Möhler, H. (2006). GABA A receptor diversity and pharmacology. *Cell and Tissue Research*, 326(2), 505–516.

CHAPTER 25

GALANIN

1. Introduction

Galanin is a neuropeptide widely distributed in the central and peripheral nervous systems. It plays diverse physiological roles including modulation of pain, mood regulation, feeding behavior, neuroprotection, and neuroendocrine function. The effects of galanin are mediated through specific G protein-coupled receptors known as galanin receptors.

2. Definition

Galanin receptors are a group of G protein-coupled receptors (GPCRs) that bind galanin and galanin-like peptides to mediate their effects on neuronal and non-neuronal tissues. They function by coupling to intracellular G proteins and triggering signaling cascades that modulate various cellular processes.

3. Classification of Galanin Receptors

There are three main subtypes of galanin receptors:

I. **GALR1 (Galanin Receptor 1)**: these are coupled to Gi/Go proteins and inhibits adenylate cyclase → which decreases cAMP

II. **GALR2 (Galanin Receptor 2):** these are coupled to Gq/11 proteins and activates phospholipase C → increases IP3 and DAG → Ca2+ mobilization and PKC activation

III. **GALR3 (Galanin Receptor 3)**: these are also coupled to Gi/Go proteins and Inhibits adenylate cyclase and regulates potassium and calcium channels.

4. Pharmacological Actions

A. **Neurotransmission Modulation**: Galanin modulates excitatory and inhibitory neurotransmitters such as serotonin, norepinephrine, dopamine, and GABA.
B. **Pain Regulation**: Antinociceptive effects via spinal and supraspinal mechanisms
C. **Feeding Behavior**: Stimulates appetite and feeding through hypothalamic pathways
D. **Neuroendocrine Effects**: it influences secretion of growth hormone, prolactin, and luteinizing hormone
E. **Neuroprotection**: it supports neuronal survival and inhibits neuroinflammation

5. Therapeutic Indications

Although currently there are no FDA-approved drugs specifically targeting galanin receptors, preclinical and early clinical studies suggest potential roles in the treatment of:

- Neuropathic Pain
- Depression and Anxiety Disorders
- Epilepsy
- Alzheimer's Disease and Neurodegeneration
- Eating Disorders and Obesity

6. Contraindications and Precautions

Because selective galanin receptor modulators are still under investigation, definitive contraindications are not fully established. However, potential issues include:

- ❖ **Mood Disorders**: Galanin can influence serotonergic and noradrenergic transmission, potentially worsening depression in certain contexts
- ❖ **Appetite Regulation**: Agents affecting GALR1/2 could lead to metabolic disturbances or weight gain
- ❖ **Hormonal Imbalance**: Effects on pituitary hormones may pose risks in endocrine disorders
- ❖ **Cardiovascular Effects**: Galanin may influence autonomic tone and vascular reactivity

7. Summary

Galanin receptors represent a promising target class for novel therapeutic strategies, particularly in neuropsychiatric and pain-related disorders. Continued research is needed to develop selective agonists and antagonists and to evaluate their safety and efficacy in clinical populations.

References

1. Lang, R., Gundlach, A. L., & Holmes, F. E. (2015). Advances in galanin receptor pharmacology: Ligands, signaling, and therapeutic potential. *Frontiers in Endocrinology*, 6, 121.
2. Branchek, T. A., Smith, K. E., Gerald, C., & Walker, M. W. (2000). Galanin receptor subtypes. *Trends in Pharmacological Sciences*, 21(3), 109–117.
3. Mitsukawa, K., Lu, X., Bartfai, T., &Hökfelt, T. (2008). Galanin, galanin receptor subtypes and depression-like behavior. *Cellular and Molecular Life Sciences*, 65(12), 1854–1861.
4. Xu, Z. Q. D., Shi, T. J. S., &Hökfelt, T. (1996). Galanin/GMAP- and galanin message-associated peptide-like immunoreactivities in the CNS: New insights from single- and double-labeling studies. *Journal of Comparative Neurology*, 369(3), 413–434.
5. Waters, S. M., Krause, J. E. (2000). Distribution of galanin receptor subtype mRNAs in the rat central nervous system. *Brain Research Molecular Brain Research*, 80(2), 165–177.

CHAPTER 26

GHRELIN

1. Introduction

Ghrelin is a peptide hormone primarily secreted by the stomach that plays a crucial role in regulating appetite, energy homeostasis, and growth hormone secretion. Its physiological effects are mediated through the ghrelin receptor, making it a significant target in metabolic, endocrine, and neurological research.

2. Definition

Ghrelin receptors, also known as Growth Hormone Secretagogue Receptors (GHS-Rs), are G protein-coupled receptors (GPCRs) that mediate the effects of ghrelin. These receptors are widely expressed in the central nervous system, especially in the hypothalamus and pituitary gland, as well as in peripheral tissues.

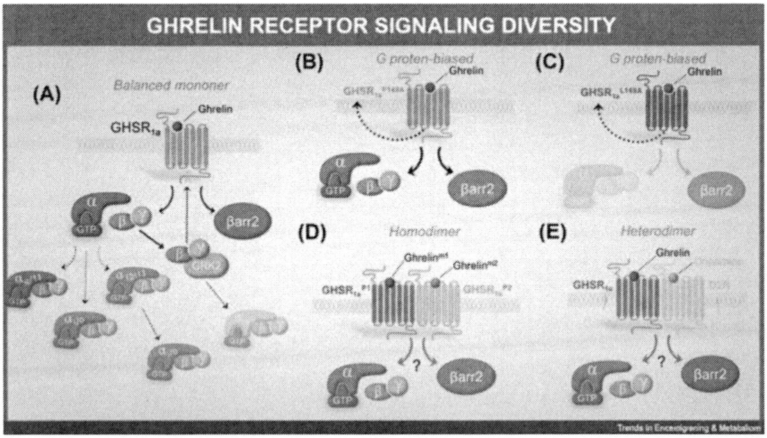

Fig. 26.1Ghrelin receptors and signailing mechanism.

3. Classification

Ghrelin receptors are primarily classified into two isoforms resulting from alternative splicing:

A. **GHS-R1a**: The functional receptor isoform that binds acylated ghrelin and activates intracellular signaling.
B. **GHS-R1b**: A truncated, non-functional isoform that does not bind ghrelin or activate G proteins; its role may be regulatory or inhibitory.

4. Pharmacological Actions

I. **Growth Hormone Secretion**: GHS-R1a stimulates the release of growth hormone from the anterior pituitary.
II. **Appetite Stimulation**: Activation in the hypothalamus increases food intake and promotes adiposity.
III. **Glucose Homeostasis**: Ghrelin influences insulin secretion and glucose metabolism.
IV. **Gastrointestinal Motility**: Enhances gastric emptying and motility.
V. **Cardiovascular Effects**: May exert cardioprotective effects, including modulation of blood pressure and cardiac output.
VI. **Neuroprotection and Cognition**: Involved in memory, learning, and neurogenesis.

5. Therapeutic Indications

While ghrelin receptor-targeted drugs are still under development, the receptor is being explored for therapeutic interventions in:

- **Cachexia and Anorexia** (e.g., cancer-related, AIDS-related)
- **Growth Hormone Deficiency**
- **Gastrointestinal Disorders** (e.g., gastroparesis)
- **Neurodegenerative Diseases** (e.g., Alzheimer's disease)
- **Obesity and Metabolic Syndrome** (using antagonists/inverse agonists)

6. Contraindications and Precautions

Although selective modulators of the ghrelin receptor are not yet widely used in clinical practice, potential contraindications and precautions may include:

- **Obesity and Diabetes**: Agonists may exacerbate hyperphagia and insulin resistance.
- **Cancer**: Ghrelin's growth-promoting effects could theoretically support tumor progression.
- **Cardiovascular Conditions**: Although generally beneficial, ghrelin's vasodilatory actions may require caution in hypotensive patients.
- **Hormone-sensitive Conditions**: Interactions with endocrine axes need monitoring in patients with hormonal imbalances.

7. Summary

Ghrelin receptors are pivotal in mediating energy balance, growth regulation, and neuroendocrine functions. Continued exploration of GHS-R1a and its pharmacology presents a promising frontier for therapeutic innovations in metabolic and neurodegenerative diseases.

References

1. Kojima, M., Hosoda, H., Date, Y., Nakazato, M., Matsuo, H., &Kangawa, K. (1999). Ghrelin is a growth-hormone-releasing acylated peptide from stomach. *Nature*, 402(6762), 656–660.
2. Howard, A. D., Feighner, S. D., Cully, D. F., et al. (1996). A receptor in pituitary and hypothalamus that functions in growth hormone release. *Science*, 273(5277), 974–977.
3. Müller, T. D., Nogueiras, R., Andermann, M. L., Andrews, Z. B., Anker, S. D., Argente, J., et al. (2015). Ghrelin. *Molecular Metabolism*, 4(6), 437–460.
4. van der Lely, A. J., Tschöp, M., Heiman, M. L., & Ghigo, E. (2004). Biological, physiological, pathophysiological, and pharmacological aspects of ghrelin. *Endocrine Reviews*, 25(3), 426–457.
5. Sun, Y., Wang, P., Zheng, H., & Smith, R. G. (2004). Ghrelin stimulation of growth hormone release and appetite is mediated through the growth hormone secretagogue receptor. *PNAS*, 101(13), 4679–4684.

CHAPTER 27

GLUCAGON RECEPTORS

1. Introduction

Glucagon is a peptide hormone produced by the alpha cells of the pancreas. It plays a central role in glucose metabolism by promoting glycogenolysis and gluconeogenesis. The physiological actions of glucagon are mediated through specific glucagon receptors, making them vital in the context of metabolic disorders like diabetes and obesity.

2. Definition

Glucagon receptors are G protein-coupled receptors (GPCRs) that specifically bind to glucagon to initiate intracellular signaling cascades. These receptors are primarily located in the liver but are also expressed in the kidneys, heart, adipose tissue, and brain.

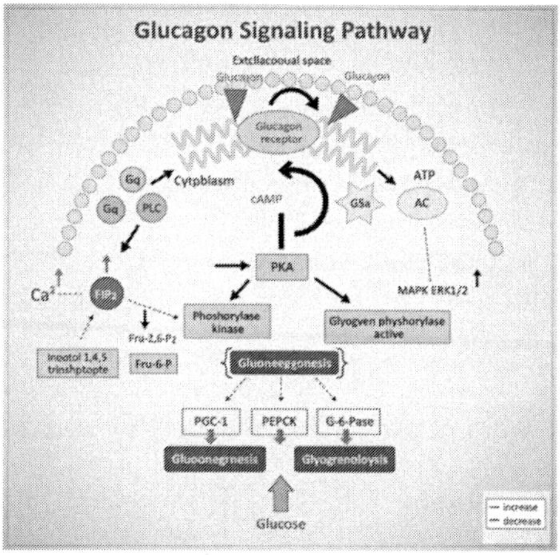

Fig.27.1Glucagon Receptorssignailing pathway.

3. Classification

The glucagon receptor belongs to the Class B (Secretin-like) family of GPCRs. It is a single member receptor with the following classification:

- **Glucagon Receptor (GCGR)**: it is activated by endogenous glucagon and belongs to Class B1 GPCRs. It is Closely related to receptors for GLP-1 and GIP (other Class B1 family members)

4. Pharacological Actions

Upon glucagon binding, the glucagon receptor activates intracellular signaling through Gs proteins, leading to:

- ❖ **Adenylate Cyclase Activation** → Increases cAMP levels → Activates Protein Kinase A (PKA)
- ❖ **Glycogenolysis**: Breakdown of glycogen to glucose in the liver
- ❖ **Gluconeogenesis**: Promotion of glucose synthesis from non-carbohydrate sources
- ❖ **Lipolysis**: Mobilization of fat stores
- ❖ **Cardiac Effects**: Positive inotropic and chronotropic effects

5. Therapeutic Indications

- **Severe Hypoglycemia:** used in emergency treatment using injectable or nasal glucagon formulations
- **Diagnostic Use**: Used during radiologic imaging (e.g., gastrointestinal tract procedures) to reduce intestinal motility
- **Obesity and Diabetes Research**: Glucagon receptor antagonists and dual agonists (e.g., GLP-1/glucagon) are under investigation for weight loss and glucose control
- **Heart Failure**: Investigational use due to glucagon's inotropic effects

6. Contraindications and Precautions

- **Pheochromocytoma**: Risk of catecholamine surge and hypertensive crisis
- **Insulinoma**: May lead to rebound hypoglycemia
- **Hypersensitivity**: Rare allergic reactions to glucagon preparations

- **Starvation or Adrenal Insufficiency**: Reduced hepatic glycogen stores can impair glucagon efficacy
- **Chronic Liver Disease**: Diminished glycogen storage may limit the response to glucagon

7. Summary

The glucagon receptor is integral to glucose and energy homeostasis and has emerged as a promising target for therapeutic interventions in metabolic and cardiovascular conditions. Continued research on receptor agonists, antagonists, and dual-acting peptides may yield novel strategies for managing diabetes, obesity, and heart failure.

References

1. Roberts, D. J., &Kraegen, E. W. (2017). The role of the glucagon receptor in energy metabolism. *Nature Reviews Endocrinology*, 13(6), 329–336.
2. Kazda, C. M., Ding, Y., Kelly, R. P., et al. (2016). Evaluation of efficacy and safety of the glucagon receptor antagonist LY2409021 in type 2 diabetes. *Diabetes Care*, 39(7), 1241–1249.
3. Müller, T. D., Finan, B., Bloom, S. R., et al. (2019). Glucagon-like peptide 1 (GLP-1). *Molecular Metabolism*, 30, 72–130.
4. Holst, J. J. (2013). The physiology of glucagon-like peptide 1. *Physiological Reviews*, 87(4), 1409–1439.
5. Perry, R. J., Shulman, G. I. (2020). Mechanistic insights into glucagon receptor signaling in liver metabolism. *Trends in Endocrinology and Metabolism*, 31(6), 476–487.

CHAPTER 28

GLYCOPROTEIN HORMONE RECEPTORS

1. Introduction

Glycoprotein hormone receptors are a specialized subset of G protein-coupled receptors (GPCRs) that mediate the physiological actions of glycoprotein hormones, including luteinizing hormone (LH), follicle-stimulating hormone (FSH), thyroid-stimulating hormone (TSH), and human chorionic gonadotropin (hCG). These hormones are key regulators of reproductive and metabolic processes, making their receptors critical targets in both diagnostic and therapeutic endocrinology.

2. Definition

Glycoprotein hormone receptors are membrane-bound receptors that specifically bind to large, heterodimeric glycoprotein hormones. They consist of a large extracellular domain responsible for ligand binding and a seven-transmembrane domain typical of GPCRs, which activates downstream signaling pathways.

3. Classification

Glycoprotein hormone receptors are classified based on their ligand specificity:

A. Luteinizing Hormone/Chorionic Gonadotropin Receptor (LHCGR)
B. Follicle-Stimulating Hormone Receptor (FSHR)
C. Thyroid-Stimulating Hormone Receptor (TSHR)

All three belong to the Class A (rhodopsin-like) GPCR family and share structural similarities, including leucine-rich repeat domains in their extracellular regions.

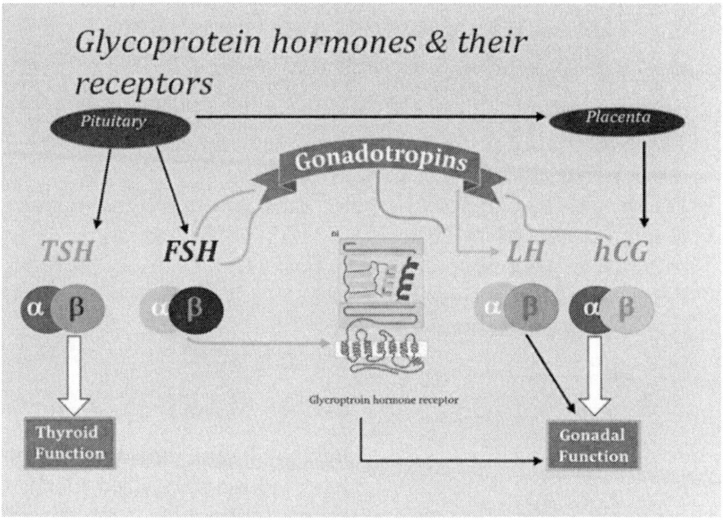

Fig. 28.1 Glycoprotein hormone receptors and function.

4. Pharmacological Actions

A. **FSHR**: Stimulates granulosa cell development and estrogen production in females; regulates spermatogenesis in males.
B. **LHCGR**: Induces ovulation and progesterone production in females; stimulates testosterone production in males.
C. **TSHR**: Promotes thyroid hormone synthesis and secretion (T3 and T4); regulates thyroid cell proliferation.

The receptors primarily signal through Gs proteins, activating adenylate cyclase → increased cAMP → activation of protein kinase A (PKA).

5. Therapeutic Indications

A. **FSHR Agonists**: Used in assisted reproductive technologies (ART), such as in vitro fertilization (e.g., recombinant FSH)
B. **LHCGR Agonists**: hCG injections to induce ovulation or testosterone production
C. **TSHR Agonists/Antagonists**: Limited clinical use, but TSH is used diagnostically in thyroid cancer monitoring

6. Contraindications and Precautions

A. **Ovarian Hyperstimulation Syndrome (OHSS)**: Risk in women treated with FSH and hCG
B. **Thyroid Disorders**: TSH analogs or alterations in TSHR activity may exacerbate hyper- or hypothyroidism
C. **Pregnancy**: Use of gonadotropins should be carefully monitored
D. **Hormone-sensitive Cancers**: Caution with gonadotropin use in patients with hormone-dependent tumors
E. **Polycystic Ovary Syndrome (PCOS)**: Patients may be at higher risk for complications during ART

7. Summary

Glycoprotein hormone receptors are vital for the regulation of reproductive and thyroid functions. Their well-characterized mechanisms and physiological relevance make them indispensable in endocrinology, reproductive medicine, and thyroid diagnostics. Future developments in receptor modulators may broaden therapeutic applications.

References

1. Ascoli, M., Fanelli, F., &Segaloff, D. L. (2002). The luteinizing hormone/chorionic gonadotropin receptor: A 2002 perspective. *Endocrine Reviews*, 23(2), 141–174.
2. Ulloa-Aguirre, A., Reiter, E., &Crepieux, P. (2011). FSH receptor signaling: Complexity of interactions and signal diversity. *Endocrinology*, 152(4), 1687–1696.
3. Latronico, A. C., &Segaloff, D. L. (2007). Insights into the function of the FSH receptor and TSH receptor from human mutations. *Molecular and Cellular Endocrinology*, 260-262, 110–118.
4. Libert, F., Lefort, A., Gerard, C., et al. (1990). Cloning, sequencing, and expression of the human thyrotropin (TSH) receptor: Evidence for constitutive activity. *EMBO Journal*, 9(11), 3475–3484.
5. Themmen, A. P. N., &Huhtaniemi, I. T. (2000). Mutations of gonadotropins and gonadotropin receptors: Elucidating the physiology and pathophysiology of pituitary-gonadal function. *Endocrine Reviews*, 21(5), 551–583.

CHAPTER 29

GONADOTROPIN RECEPTORS

1. Introduction

Gonadotropin receptors are integral membrane proteins that mediate the physiological actions of the glycoprotein hormones—luteinizing hormone (LH), follicle-stimulating hormone (FSH), and human chorionic gonadotropin (hCG). These hormones play essential roles in reproductive function, including gametogenesis, steroidogenesis, and gonadal development. The receptors are members of the G protein-coupled receptor (GPCR) superfamily.

2. Definition

Gonadotropin receptors are specific GPCRs that bind gonadotropins to activate intracellular signaling pathways essential for reproductive processes. They include the luteinizing hormone/choriogonadotropin receptor (LHCGR) and the follicle-stimulating hormone receptor (FSHR), both of which share a common seven-transmembrane domain structure.

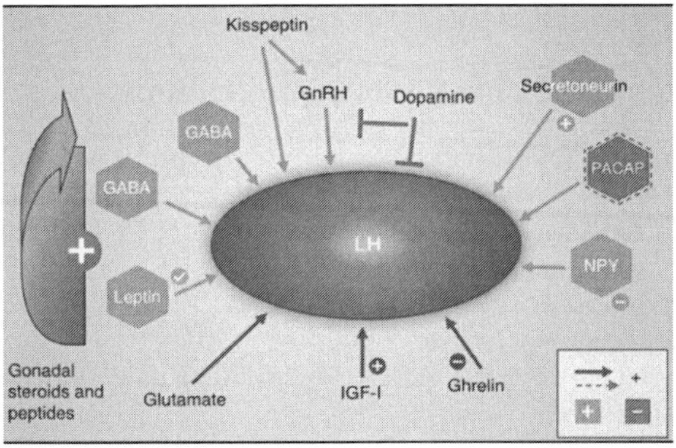

Fig. 29.1 Gonadotropin receptors and Pharmacological actions.

3. Classification

Gonadotropin receptors are classified into two primary types:

A. **Luteinizing Hormone/Chorionic Gonadotropin Receptor (LHCGR)**
   - Binds both LH and hCG
   - Expressed in Leydig cells (testes) and theca/luteal cells (ovaries)

B. **Follicle-Stimulating Hormone Receptor (FSHR)**
   - Binds FSH
   - Expressed in granulosa cells (ovaries) and Sertoli cells (testes)

These receptors belong to the Class A (rhodopsin-like) GPCR family.

4. Pharmacological Actions

Activation of these receptors by gonadotropins results in:

A. **LHCGR**: Stimulates production of sex steroids (testosterone, progesterone), induces ovulation, and supports corpus luteum maintenance.

B. **FSHR**: Promotes follicular maturation, estrogen synthesis, and spermatogenesis.

Signaling primarily involves the Gs protein–mediated activation of adenylate cyclase → increased cyclic AMP (cAMP) → protein kinase A (PKA) activation.

5. Therapeutic Indications

I. **Infertility Treatment**: Recombinant or urinary-derived FSH and hCG are used to stimulate ovulation and spermatogenesis.

II. **Assisted Reproductive Technologies (ART)**: Used in controlled ovarian stimulation protocols

III. **Hypogonadotropic Hypogonadism**: Gonadotropin therapy restores reproductive function

IV. **Delayed Puberty**: In selected cases, hCG or FSH may be used to initiate puberty

6. Contraindications and Precautions

- **Ovarian Hyperstimulation Syndrome (OHSS)**: Risk in women undergoing fertility treatments
- **Pregnancy**: Gonadotropin administration is contraindicated
- **Hormone-sensitive Tumors**: Contraindicated in patients with breast, ovarian, or uterine cancers
- **Primary Gonadal Failure**: Ineffectiveness due to lack of functional gonadal tissue
- **Uncontrolled Thyroid or Adrenal Disorders**: These should be corrected prior to gonadotropin therapy

7. Summary

Gonadotropin receptors are essential regulators of human reproduction. Advances in receptor pharmacology and the development of recombinant gonadotropins have significantly improved the management of infertility. Continued research into receptor mutations and signaling dynamics holds promise for more targeted therapies.

References

1. Simoni, M., Gromoll, J., &Nieschlag, E. (1997). The follicle-stimulating hormone receptor: Biochemistry, molecular biology, physiology, and pathophysiology. *Endocrine Reviews*, 18(6), 739–773.
2. Ascoli, M., Fanelli, F., &Segaloff, D. L. (2002). The luteinizing hormone/chorionic gonadotropin receptor: A 2002 perspective. *Endocrine Reviews*, 23(2), 141–174.
3. Themmen, A. P. N., &Huhtaniemi, I. T. (2000). Mutations of gonadotropins and gonadotropin receptors: Elucidating the physiology and pathophysiology of pituitary-gonadal function. *Endocrine Reviews*, 21(5), 551–583.
4. Ulloa-Aguirre, A., Reiter, E., &Crepieux, P. (2011). FSH receptor signaling: Complexity of interactions and signal diversity. *Endocrinology*, 152(4), 1687–1696.
5. Latronico, A. C., &Segaloff, D. L. (2007). Insights into the function of the FSH receptor and TSH receptor from human mutations. *Molecular and Cellular Endocrinology*, 260-262, 110–118.

CHAPTER 30

HISTAMINE RECEPTORS

1. Introduction

Histamine is a biogenic amine that plays a central role in immune responses, gastric acid secretion, neurotransmission, and inflammation. Its actions are mediated through four types of histamine receptors (H1, H2, H3, and H4), which are all G protein-coupled receptors (GPCRs). These receptors are distributed in various tissues and elicit diverse physiological and pathological effects.

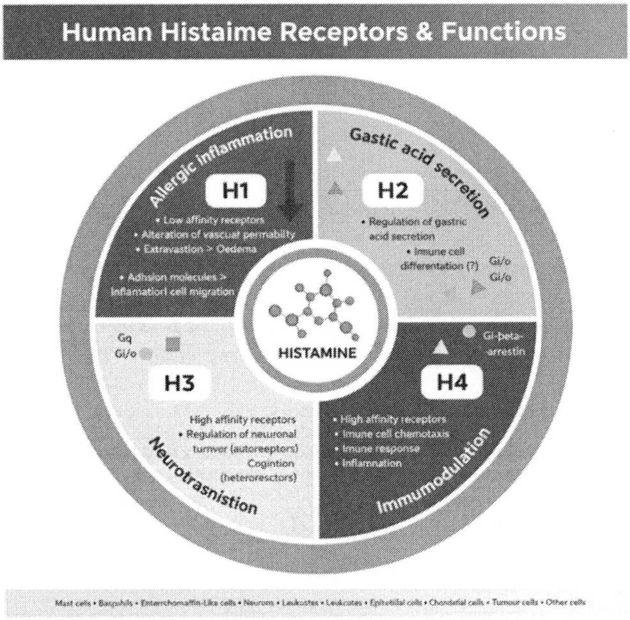

Fig. 30.1 Histamine Receptors types and functions.

2. Definition

Histamine receptors are a group of GPCRs that mediate the biological effects of histamine. Each receptor subtype is linked to specific intracellular signaling pathways and biological responses. Their activation or inhibition forms the basis of several therapeutic interventions.

3. Classification

Histamine receptors are classified into four main subtypes:

A. **H1 Receptors**
   - Located in smooth muscle, endothelium, and the brain
   - Mediates allergic responses, vasodilation, and wakefulness

B. **H2 Receptors**
   - Primarily in gastric parietal cells, heart, and brain
   - Stimulates gastric acid secretion and modulates cardiac function

C. **H3 Receptors**
   - Found in the central nervous system (CNS)
   - Functions as autoreceptors and heteroreceptors regulating neurotransmitter release

D. **H4 Receptors**
   - Expressed in bone marrow and white blood cells
   - Involved in chemotaxis and immune modulation

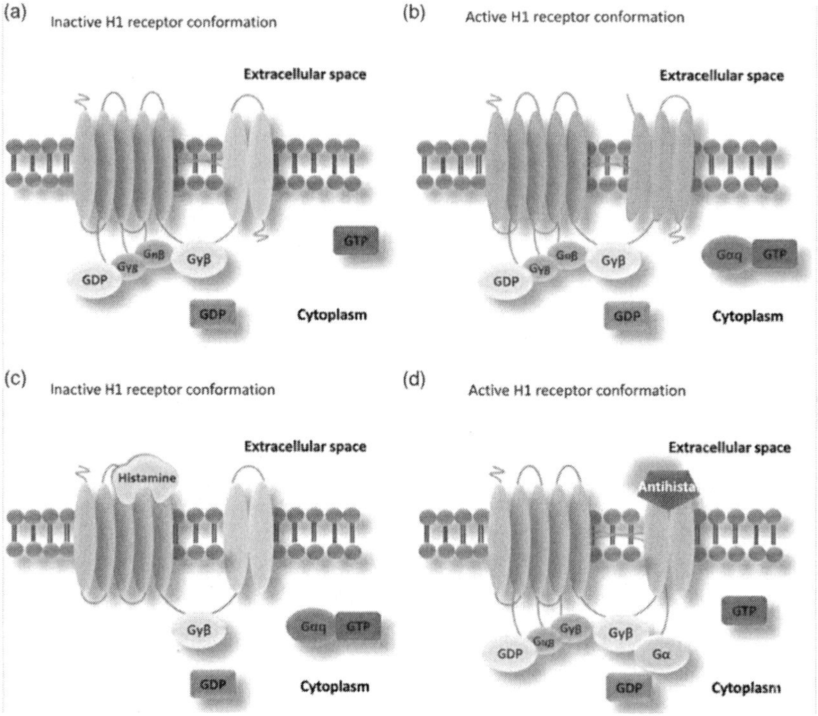

Fig. 30.2 Histamine Receptors activation amd actions.

4. Pharmacological Actions

A. **H1 Receptor Activation**: it increases vascular permeability, bronchoconstriction, and sensory nerve stimulation and also involved in allergic reactions and inflammation

B. **H2 Receptor Activation**
   - It Stimulates gastric acid secretion
   - It Promotes smooth muscle relaxation and positive chronotropic effects

C. **H3 Receptor Activation**
   - It Inhibits histamine and other neurotransmitter release (dopamine, acetylcholine)
   - It Modulates sleep-wake cycles and cognition

D. **H4 Receptor Activation**
   - It Regulates immune cell chemotaxis and cytokine production

5. Therapeutic Indications

A. **H1 Antagonists (Antihistamines)**: they Used in allergic rhinitis, urticaria, anaphylaxis, and motion sicknessExamples: Diphenhydramine, Loratadine
B. **H2 Antagonists**: they used in peptic ulcer disease, GERD, and Zollinger-Ellison syndrome. Examples: Ranitidine, Famotidine
C. **H3 Receptor Modulators**: Used as investigational agents for narcolepsy, ADHD, and cognitive disorders
D. **H4 Receptor Antagonists**: they are under research for autoimmune diseases, asthma, and pruritus

6. Contraindications and Precautions

I. **H1 Antagonists**: First-generation antihistamines cause sedation; contraindicated in glaucoma and prostatic hypertrophy
II. **H2 Antagonists**: Caution in hepatic and renal impairment; potential drug interactions via cytochrome P450 inhibition
III. **H3/H4 Agents**: Safety profiles under evaluation; not widely approved for clinical use

Summary

Histamine receptors are critical mediators of numerous physiological processes, from allergic responses to neurotransmission and immune regulation. Therapeutic targeting of these receptors has significantly improved the management of allergic, gastric, and inflammatory disorders. Ongoing research into H3 and H4 receptor modulation holds promise for novel therapeutic avenues.

References

1. Parsons, M. E., &Ganellin, C. R. (2006). Histamine and its receptors. *British Journal of Pharmacology*, 147(S1), S127–S135.
2. Thurmond, R. L., Gelfand, E. W., & Dunford, P. J. (2008). The role of histamine H1 and H4 receptors in allergic inflammation: The search for new antihistamines. *Nature Reviews Drug Discovery*, 7(1), 41–53.
3. Haas, H. L., Sergeeva, O. A., & Selbach, O. (2008). Histamine in the nervous system. *Physiological Reviews*, 88(3), 1183–1241.

4. Panula, P., Chazot, P. L., Cowart, M., et al. (2015). International Union of Basic and Clinical Pharmacology. XCVIII. Histamine receptors. *Pharmacological Reviews*, 67(3), 601–655.
5. Leurs, R., Chazot, P. L., Shenton, F. C., Lim, H. D., & de Esch, I. J. P. (2009). Molecular and biochemical pharmacology of the histamine H4 receptor. *British Journal of Pharmacology*, 157(1), 14–23.

Clinical Importance

Histamine H_1/H_2 receptors — Anaphylaxis and antihistamine pharmacology adjunct to epinephrineVignette idea:

Patient with bee sting anaphylaxis treated with IM epinephrine and adjunct H_1 antihistamines; explain histamine receptor subtypes, their systemic effects (vasodilation, bronchospasm, gastric acid), and why antihistamines are supportive (not primary) in anaphylaxis.

CHAPTER 31

KISSPEPTIN RECEPTORS

1. Introduction

Kisspeptin receptors (KISS1R), also known as GPR54, are a group of G protein-coupled receptors (GPCRs) that bind kisspeptins—peptides derived from the KISS1 gene. These receptors play a crucial role in the regulation of the hypothalamic-pituitary-gonadal (HPG) axis and are essential for the initiation of puberty, reproductive hormone secretion, and fertility. Recent research has also implicated kisspeptin signaling in cancer biology and metabolic regulation.

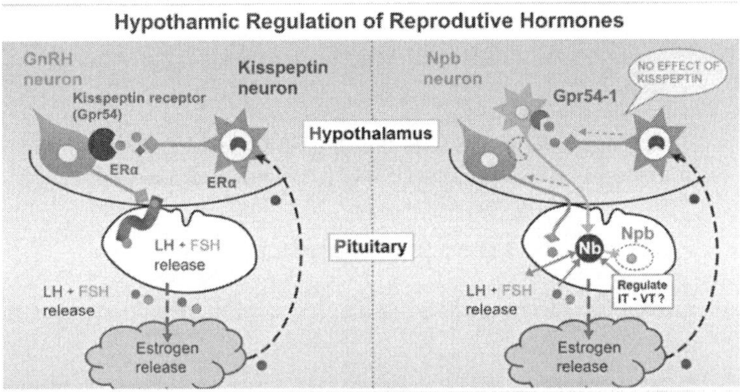

Fig. 31.1 Kisspeptin receptors and actions in reproduction system.

2. Definition

Kisspeptin receptors (KISS1R or GPR54) are GPCRs that mediate the biological actions of kisspeptins. These receptors are primarily expressed in the hypothalamus, placenta, and reproductive organs. They initiate intracellular signaling cascades through Gq/11 proteins upon ligand binding.

3. Classification

Kisspeptin receptors belong to the Class A (rhodopsin-like) family of GPCRs. Currently, only one functional receptor subtype has been identified in humans:

A. **KISS1R (GPR54)**
   - High-affinity receptor for kisspeptins (mainly kisspeptin-10, -13, and -54)
   - Coupled to Gq/11 proteins leading to phospholipase C activation

4. Pharmacological Actions

Kisspeptin binding to KISS1R activates the Gq/11 signaling pathway, resulting in:

- Activation of phospholipase C (PLC)
- Increase in inositol trisphosphate (IP3) and diacylglycerol (DAG)
- Intracellular calcium release and activation of protein kinase C (PKC)
- Modulation of GnRH (Gonadotropin-releasing hormone) neuron activity

These actions ultimately stimulate the release of luteinizing hormone (LH) and follicle-stimulating hormone (FSH) from the anterior pituitary.

5. Therapeutic Indications

Kisspeptin and its receptor are being explored as therapeutic targets in the following areas:

A. **Reproductive Disorders**
   - Diagnosis and management of delayed puberty, hypogonadotropic hypogonadism
   - Infertility treatment through kisspeptin-induced LH/FSH stimulation

B. **Assisted Reproduction**
   - Used to safely trigger oocyte maturation in IVF protocols, reducing risk of ovarian hyperstimulation syndrome (OHSS)

C. **Cancer Research**
   - ❖ Investigated for their tumor-suppressive roles in breast, melanoma, and pancreatic cancers

D. **Metabolic Disorders**
   - ❖ Implicated in energy balance and insulin sensitivity (preclinical stage)

6. Contraindications and Precautions

Although kisspeptin-based therapies are generally well tolerated, the following considerations are important:

A. **Pregnancy**: Use in pregnancy is not well studied and may affect placental function

B. **Hormone-sensitive Cancers**: Stimulation of gonadotropins may be contraindicated in estrogen- or androgen-sensitive tumors

C. **Cardiovascular Risk**: Hypothetical risk due to kisspeptin-induced vasoconstriction and changes in vascular tone

D. **Prepubertal Children**: Not suitable unless used under strict endocrine supervision

7. Summary

Kisspeptin receptors represent a pivotal control point in the regulation of the reproductive axis. Their role in fertility, puberty, and potentially tumor suppression underscores their biomedical importance. As research progresses, KISS1R may become a valuable target for both diagnostic and therapeutic innovations in reproductive endocrinology and oncology.

References

1. Oakley, A. E., Clifton, D. K., & Steiner, R. A. (2009). Kisspeptin signaling in the brain. *Endocrine Reviews*, 30(6), 713–743.
2. Seminara, S. B., Messager, S., Chatzidaki, E. E., et al. (2003). The GPR54 gene as a regulator of puberty. *New England Journal of Medicine*, 349(17), 1614–1627.
3. Jayasena, C. N., Abbara, A., Comninos, A. N., et al. (2014). Kisspeptin-54 triggers egg maturation in women undergoing IVF. *Journal of Clinical Investigation*, 124(8), 3667–3677.
4. Curtis, V. M., & Shah, A. H. (2008). Kisspeptins and the regulation of the HPG axis. *Reproduction*, 135(6), 721–729.

5. Mead, E. J., Maguire, J. J., Kuc, R. E., & Davenport, A. P. (2007). Kisspeptins: A multifunctional peptide system with a role in reproduction, cancer, and the cardiovascular system. *British Journal of Pharmacology*, 151(8), 1143–1153.

CHAPTER 32

LEUKOTRIENE RECEPTORS

1. Introduction

Leukotriene receptors are a subgroup of G protein-coupled receptors (GPCRs) that bind leukotrienes—lipid mediators derived from arachidonic acid via the 5-lipoxygenase pathway. These receptors play crucial roles in inflammatory and allergic responses, particularly in asthma, allergic rhinitis, and cardiovascular diseases. Targeting leukotriene receptors has emerged as an effective therapeutic approach in managing chronic inflammatory conditions.

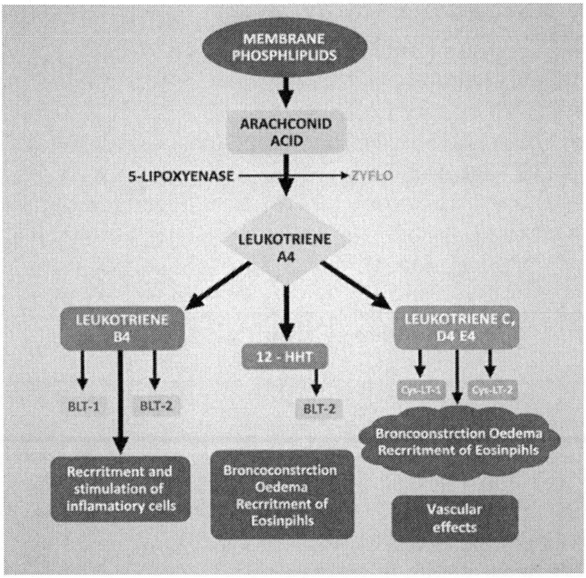

Fig. 32.1 Leukotriene synthesis and subtypes of leukotrienes receptors.

2. Definition

Leukotriene receptors are membrane-bound GPCRs that mediate the biological actions of leukotrienes, including bronchoconstriction, vascular permeability, and recruitment of immune cells. They are primarily expressed in immune cells, smooth muscle, and the respiratory tract.

3. Classification

Leukotriene receptors are primarily classified into two main subtypes based on their ligand specificity:

A. **Cysteinyl Leukotriene Receptors (CysLTRs)**
   a. **CysLT1 receptor**
      - High affinity for LTD4 > LTC4 > LTE4
      - Located in bronchial smooth muscle, eosinophils, and mast cells
   b. **CysLT2 receptor**
      - High affinity for LTC4 = LTD4 > LTE4
      - Found in endothelial cells and heart

B. **BLT Receptors (Bind Leukotriene B4)**
   a. **BLT1 receptor**
      - High affinity for LTB4
      - Expressed in neutrophils and other leukocytes
   b. **BLT2 receptor**
      - Low affinity for LTB4, broader ligand recognition
      - Found in epithelial cells and tissues not involved in classic inflammation

4. Pharmacological Actions

Leukotriene receptors mediate diverse pro-inflammatory actions depending on the receptor subtype:

A. **CysLT1 and CysLT2 Receptors**
   - Bronchoconstriction
   - Increased vascular permeability
   - Mucus secretion in airways
   - Eosinophil recruitment

B. **BLT1 and BLT2 Receptors**
   - Chemotaxis and activation of neutrophils

- o Promotion of inflammatory cytokine release

Pharmacological modulation includes antagonism of these receptors using drugs like montelukast, which inhibits CysLT1-mediated responses.

5. Therapeutic Indications

Leukotriene receptor antagonists and inhibitors have various clinical applications:

- **Asthma and Allergic Rhinitis**: Montelukast and zafirlukast as oral anti-asthmatic agents
- **Exercise-Induced Bronchoconstriction**: Montelukast provides prophylactic protection
- **Aspirin-Exacerbated Respiratory Disease (AERD)**: Effective symptom control in NSAID-sensitive asthma
- **Urticaria and Atopic Dermatitis**: Used off-label for inflammation control

6. Contraindications and Precautions

Although leukotriene receptor antagonists are generally well tolerated, certain precautions apply:

- **Liver Dysfunction**: Zileuton may elevate liver enzymes and should be avoided in hepatic impairment
- **Neuropsychiatric Effects**: Rare but serious side effects include agitation, depression, and suicidal ideation (notably with montelukast)
- **Hypersensitivity**: Reactions such as Churg-Strauss syndrome may develop after corticosteroid withdrawal
- **Pregnancy and Lactation**: Use only if benefits outweigh risks; safety not fully established

7. Summary

Leukotriene receptors are key players in mediating inflammatory and allergic responses. Their selective antagonism has led to effective therapies, particularly in respiratory and immune-mediated diseases. Ongoing research continues to explore their role in cardiovascular, dermatological, and cancer-related inflammation.

References

1. Peters-Golden, M., & Henderson, W. R. (2007). Leukotrienes. *New England Journal of Medicine*, 357(18), 1841–1854.
2. Singh, D., & Papi, A. (2010). The role of leukotriene receptor antagonists in asthma management. *Therapeutic Advances in Respiratory Disease*, 4(3), 173–185.
3. Capra, V., Rovati, G. E., Mangano, P., Buccellati, C., Murphy, R. C., & Sala, A. (2007). Transcellular biosynthesis of eicosanoids. *Pharmacological Reports*, 59(1), 75–83.
4. Drazen, J. M., Israel, E., & O'Byrne, P. M. (1999). Treatment of asthma with drugs modifying the leukotriene pathway. *New England Journal of Medicine*, 340(3), 197–206.
5. Rovati, G. E., Capra, V., & Folco, G. (2007). The cysteinyl leukotriene receptors and their antagonists. *Pharmacology & Therapeutics*, 116(3), 429–455.

CHAPTER 33

MELANIN RECEPTORS

1. Introduction

Melanin receptors, primarily known as melanocortin receptors (MCRs), are G protein-coupled receptors that mediate the physiological actions of melanocortins, a group of peptides derived from pro-opiomelanocortin (POMC), such as α-MSH (alpha-melanocyte-stimulating hormone), β-MSH, and ACTH. These receptors regulate diverse functions, including pigmentation, energy homeostasis, adrenal function, sexual behavior, and inflammation.

2. Definition

Melanin receptors refer to the melanocortin receptor family, a group of GPCRs that respond to melanocortin peptides. They are involved in melanin synthesis, endocrine signaling, appetite regulation, and immune modulation.

3. Classification

There are five known melanocortin receptors, classified as follows:

A. **MC1R (Melanocortin 1 Receptor)**: Primarily involved in skin and hair pigmentation
B. **MC2R (Melanocortin 2 Receptor)**: Also known as ACTH receptor; regulates adrenal steroidogenesis
C. **MC3R (Melanocortin 3 Receptor)**: Involved in energy homeostasis and feeding behavior
D. **MC4R (Melanocortin 4 Receptor)**: Critical regulator of appetite and energy expenditure
E. **MC5R (Melanocortin 5 Receptor)**: Associated with exocrine gland function and lipid metabolism

4. Pharmacological Actions

Melanin receptors primarily signal via Gs proteins, stimulating adenylate cyclase, leading to increased cyclic AMP (cAMP) levels and activation of downstream PKA pathways. Actions include:

i. **MC1R**: Stimulates eumelanin production in melanocytes, providing photoprotection
ii. **MC2R**: Mediates ACTH-induced cortisol release from adrenal cortex
iii. **MC3R and MC4R**: Regulate energy balance, food intake, and leptin sensitivity
iv. **MC5R**: Influences sebaceous gland function and immune responses

5. Therapeutic Indications

Melanin/melanocortin receptors are targeted in a variety of clinical conditions:

1. **MC1R**: Pigmentation disorders, sunless tanning agents
2. **MC2R**: Treatment of adrenal insufficiency (e.g., congenital adrenal hyperplasia)
3. **MC4R**: Obesity treatment (e.g., setmelanotide for genetic obesity disorders)
4. **MC3R and MC5R**: Investigated for metabolic syndromes and inflammatory diseases

6. Contraindications and Precautions

Precautions with melanin receptor-targeting therapies:

- **Hormonal Disorders**: MC2R activation can affect cortisol homeostasis, leading to hypercortisolism or adrenal insufficiency
- **Cardiovascular Conditions**: MC4R agonists may cause increases in blood pressure and heart rate
- **Pregnancy and Lactation**: Safety data is limited; avoid unless necessary
- **Hyperpigmentation Risk**: MC1R agonists can cause unwanted pigmentation changes

7. Summary

Melanin receptors, through their widespread physiological roles, serve as important targets in endocrine, dermatological, and metabolic disorders. Continued research into receptor-selective agonists and antagonists offers promising avenues for therapeutic innovations in obesity, adrenal dysfunction, and pigmentary conditions.

References

1. Mountjoy, K. G., Robbins, L. S., Mortrud, M. T., & Cone, R. D. (1992). The cloning of a family of genes that encode the melanocortin receptors. *Science*, 257(5074), 1248–1251.
2. Gantz, I., & Fong, T. M. (2003). The melanocortin system. *American Journal of Physiology-Endocrinology and Metabolism*, 284(3), E468–E474.
3. Millington, G. W. (2006). The role of proopiomelanocortin (POMC) neurones in feeding behaviour. *Nutrition & Metabolism*, 3(1), 18.
4. Kühnen, P., Clément, K., Wiegand, S., et al. (2016). Proopiomelanocortin deficiency treated with a melanocortin-4 receptor agonist. *New England Journal of Medicine*, 375(3), 240–246.
5. Wikberg, J. E., &Mutulis, F. (2008). Targeting melanocortin receptors in disease. *Trends in Pharmacological Sciences*, 29(7), 350–357.

CHAPTER 34

MELATONIN RECEPTORS

1. Introduction

Melatonin receptors are a subclass of G protein-coupled receptors (GPCRs) that mediate the effects of melatonin, a neurohormone secreted primarily by the pineal gland. Melatonin plays a crucial role in the regulation of circadian rhythms, sleep-wake cycles, seasonalreproduction, and antioxidative defense. Understanding the biology and pharmacology of melatonin receptors is essential for developing therapies targeting sleep disorders, depression, cancer, and neurodegenerative diseases.

2. Definition

Melatonin receptors are high-affinity, GPCRs that bind melatonin and mediate its physiological effects. They are embedded in the cell membrane and translate extracellular melatonin signals into intracellular biochemical events.

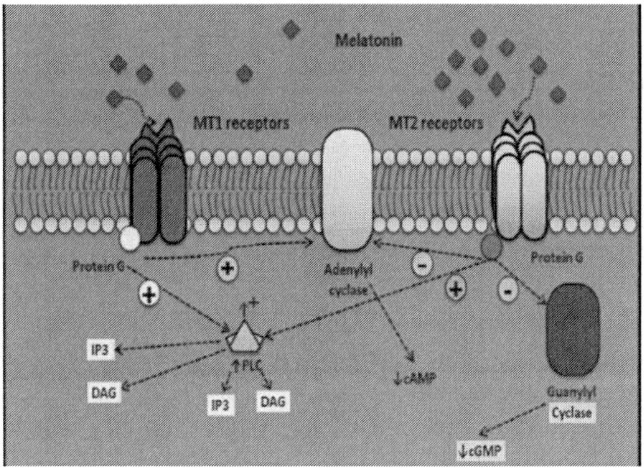

Fig. 34.1 Melatonin receptors subtypes and actions.

3. Classification

Melatonin receptors are classified into two main subtypes in mammals:

A. **MT1 (Mel1a or MTNR1A)**: Predominantly expressed in the brain, especially in the suprachiasmatic nucleus (SCN), and peripheral tissues. Regulates circadian rhythms and inhibits neuronal firing in the SCN.
B. **MT2 (Mel1b or MTNR1B):**
   - ❖ Expressed in the retina and other peripheral tissues.
   - ❖ Involved in phase-shifting circadian rhythms, sleep induction, and immune modulation.

A third receptor, **MT3**, originally described in some non-mammalian species, is now recognized as quinone reductase 2 (QR2), with less direct evidence of melatonin binding.

4. Pharmacological Actions

Melatonin receptors mediate physiological responses by coupling to Gi/o proteins, resulting in:

- ❖ Inhibition of adenylate cyclase → decreased cAMP levels
- ❖ Activation of potassium channels and inhibition of calcium channels
- ❖ Modulation of intracellular signaling pathways including PKC, MAPK, and PI3K/Akt

These actions lead to:

- ❖ Sleep induction and regulation of circadian rhythms
- ❖ Reduction in neuronal excitability
- ❖ Modulation of immune response
- ❖ Antioxidant effects and regulation of cell proliferation

5. Therapeutic Indications

Drugs targeting melatonin receptors are approved or under development for several clinical conditions:

- **Insomnia and Circadian Rhythm Disorders**
  - Ramelteon (MT1/MT2 agonist) for sleep-onset insomnia

    - Melatonin supplements for jet lag and delayed sleep phase syndrome
- **Depression and Seasonal Affective Disorder (SAD)**
    - Agomelatine (MT1/MT2 agonist and 5-HT2C antagonist) used as an antidepressant
- **Cancer**: Melatonin shows antiproliferative and pro-apoptotic effects via receptor-mediated pathways
- **Neurodegenerative Diseases**: Investigational use in Alzheimer's and Parkinson's disease for neuroprotection

6. Contraindications and Precautions

Use of melatonin receptor agonists or melatonin supplements should consider the following precautions:

- **Pregnancy and Lactation**: Limited safety data; avoid unless clearly needed
- **Autoimmune Disorders**: Caution due to potential immunomodulatory effects
- **Liver Impairment**: Dose adjustments may be necessary
- **Concomitant Use with Sedatives**: Risk of enhanced CNS depression
- **Endocrine Disorders**: Melatonin may interfere with reproductive hormone regulation

7. Summary

Melatonin receptors play a critical role in maintaining circadian physiology and have therapeutic potential in treating sleep disorders, mood disturbances, and neurodegenerative diseases. Continued research and development of selective melatonin receptor ligands offer promising avenues for precision therapeutics.

References

1. Dubocovich, M. L., Delagrange, P., Krause, D. N., Sugden, D., Cardinali, D. P., & Olcese, J. (2010). International Union of Basic and Clinical Pharmacology. LXXV. Nomenclature, classification, and pharmacology of G protein-coupled melatonin receptors. *Pharmacological Reviews*, 62(3), 343–380.

2. Hardeland, R. (2009). Melatonin: Signaling mechanisms of a pleiotropic agent. *BioFactors*, 35(2), 183–192.
3. Zawilska, J. B., & Skene, D. J. (2009). Arendt J. Physiology and pharmacology of melatonin in relation to biological rhythms. *Pharmacological Reports*, 61(3), 383–410.
4. Srinivasan, V., Spence, D. W., Pandi-Perumal, S. R., et al. (2010). Melatonin, environmental light, and breast cancer. *Breast Cancer Research and Treatment*, 115(2), 439–448.
5. Cardinali, D. P., Furio, A. M., & Reyes, M. P. (2005). Clinical perspectives for the use of melatonin as a chronobiotic and cytoprotective agent. *Annals of the New York Academy of Sciences*, 1057(1), 327–336.

CHAPTER 35

THE COMPLEXITY OF METABOTROPIC GLUTAMATE RECEPTORS

Introduction

Glutamate is the primary excitatory neurotransmitter in the vertebrate central nervous system (CNS), responsible for approximately 70% of all synaptic signaling. Its actions are mediated by two distinct super-families of receptors: ionotropic (iGluRs), which are ligand-gated ion channels mediating fast synaptic transmission, and Metabotropic Glutamate Receptors (mGluRs).

mGluRs are a family of eight subtypes of G-Protein Coupled Receptors (GPCRs). Unlike iGluRs, mGluRs do not directly form ion channels. Instead, they operate through diverse intracellular signaling cascades, providing a crucial, slower, and more modulatory layer of control over synaptic strength, plasticity, and neuronal excitability. Their widespread distribution throughout the brain—from the cortex and hippocampus to the cerebellum and basal ganglia—underscores their vital roles in learning, memory, mood, movement, and pain perception. Due to their modulatory nature and varied signaling outputs, mGluRs have become one of the most promising, yet challenging, targets for novel therapeutics aimed at neurological and psychiatric disorders.

I can certainly summarize the classifications, pharmacological actions, and indications of Metabotropic Glutamate Receptors (mGluRs) based on the Canvas document, and provide context on general pharmacological contraindications.

I. Classification and Mechanisms

The eight mGluR subtypes are categorized into three groups based on their G-protein coupling and primary cellular location/effect:

Group	Subtypes	Coupled G-Protein	Cellular Location	Primary Action
Group I		(Activatory)	Post-synaptic	**Excitatory/Modulatory:** Activates, leading to release and intracellular surge. Contributes to long-term potentiation (LTP).
Group II		(Inhibitory)	Pre- and Post-synaptic	**Inhibitory Autoreceptor:** Inhibits Adenylyl Cyclase (AC), decreasing and activity. Reduces glutamate release.
Group III		(Inhibitory)	Primarily Pre-synaptic	**Inhibitory Autoreceptor:** Shares the same inhibitory mechanism as Group II, providing negative feedback on neurotransmitter release.

II. Pharmacological Actions

Due to the risk of side effects from broad-acting orthosteric drugs (binding the main glutamate site), modern mGluR pharmacology focuses on allosteric modulation:

Drug Class	Binding Site	Effect on Receptor	Therapeutic Rationale
Positive Allosteric Modulators (PAMs)	Allosteric (non-orthosteric) site on the mGluRdimer.	**Enhances Efficacy:** Increases the receptor's sensitivity or maximum response to endogenous glutamate.	Acts as a 'volume knob' to subtly boost a weakened inhibitory or modulatory signal only when the natural neurotransmitter is present, maintaining physiological control.

Negative Allosteric Modulators (NAMs)	Allosteric (non-orthosteric) site on the mGluR dimer.	**Decreases Efficacy:** Reduces the receptor's sensitivity or maximum response to endogenous glutamate.	Acts as a 'volume knob' to subtly reduce an overactive excitatory signal or pathway.

III. Indications (Clinical Applications)

mGluRs are targeted to re-balance dysfunctional neuronal circuits implicated in various CNS disorders:

mGluR Target Group	Indication / Condition	Therapeutic Goal
(Group I)	Fragile X Syndrome (FXS), Anxiety/Depression	NAMs are used to reduce exaggerated downstream signaling and normalize hyper-excited states.
(Group II)	Schizophrenia, Anxiety	PAMs (or agonists) are used to enhance the inhibitory autoreceptor function, reducing excessive glutamatergic drive (hyperexcitation) associated with these conditions.
(Group III)	Parkinson's Disease	PAMs are used to suppress hyperactivity in the basal ganglia, thereby improving motor function.

IV. Contraindications

While the Canvas document does not specify contraindications for currently marketed mGluR drugs (as many are still in development), general pharmacological principles suggest the following considerations, particularly for broad-acting agents:

- **Group I Agonists (e.g., mGluR5 Agonists):** Due to their role in increasing and excitability, these could be contraindicated in patients with epilepsy or seizures or conditions characterized by excitotoxicity (excessive neuronal activation leading to cell death).

- **Group II/III Antagonists (e.g., mGluR2 Antagonists):** Since these receptors normally *inhibit* glutamate release, blocking them would *increase* overall glutamate signaling. They would likely be contraindicated in patients prone to psychosis or mania, where excessive glutamatergic activity is often a factor.
- **Polypharmacy:** As with all CNS-acting agents, co-administration with other drugs that affect glutamate or -protein signaling (e.g., antipsychotics, mood stabilizers) requires caution and may be relatively contraindicated until safety profiles are established.

Structural Features: The Venus Flytrap Design

mGluRs belong to Family C of the GPCR super-family, a structural distinction that separates them from the more common Family A GPCRs (like adrenergic or muscarinic receptors). Their unique structure is critical to their function:

1. Obligate Dimerization: All mGluRs function as non-covalently linked dimers. Ligand binding at one protomer can influence the activity of the other, enabling complex allosteric regulation.
2. The Venus Flytrap (VFT) Domain: The large N-terminal extracellular domain is highly characteristic. It resembles a two-lobed structure, often termed the VFT domain. Glutamate binds within the cleft between these two lobes. When glutamate binds, the lobes close, causing a conformational change that propagates through the transmembrane domain to the intracellular G-protein binding site.
3. Cysteine-Rich Domain (CRD): This domain links the VFT to the transmembrane helices. It is highly structured and helps transmit the conformational change initiated by the VFT closing.

Functional Classification and Signal Transduction

The eight mGluR subtypes (mGluR1 to mGluR8) are classified into three functional groups based on their amino acid sequence homology, coupled G-protein, and subsequent intracellular signaling pathways.

Group I mGluRs (mGluR1 and mGluR5)

Coupled G-Protein: G_q/G_11 (Activatory)

Mechanism: Group I mGluRs are typically located post-synaptically and are often found near ionotropic receptors. Activation of these receptors engages the G_qsignaling cascade:

1. The activated G_q protein activates Phospholipase C (PLC).
2. PLC hydrolyzes the membrane phospholipid phosphatidylinositol bisphosphate (PIP_2) into two critical second messengers:
    - Inositol Trisphosphate (IP_3): Binds to receptors on the endoplasmic reticulum, triggering the release of intracellular calcium ions (Ca^2+). This Ca^2+ surge is essential for neuronal plasticity and excitability.
    - Diacylglycerol (DAG): Remains in the membrane and activates Protein Kinase C (PKC), which then phosphorylates various downstream targets.

Overall Function: These receptors are generally excitatory or modulatory, often enhancing other signaling pathways and contributing significantly to long-term potentiation (LTP)—the cellular basis for learning and memory.

Group II mGluRs (mGluR2 and mGluR3) and Group III mGluRs (mGluR4, 6, 7, 8)

Coupled G-Protein: G_i/G_o (Inhibitory)

Mechanism: Both Group II and Group III share the same primary inhibitory signaling pathway:

1. The activated G_i protein inhibits the enzyme Adenylyl Cyclase (AC).
2. Inhibition of AC leads to a decrease in the production of cyclic AMP (cAMP).
3. Reduced cAMP levels decrease the activity of Protein Kinase A (PKA), leading to reduced phosphorylation of various cellular targets, including ion channels and transcription factors.

Overall Function (Groups II and III): These groups primarily act as autoreceptors located pre-synaptically. By being situated on the terminal of the glutamate-releasing neuron, their activation reduces neurotransmitter release. This mechanism provides negative feedback, acting as a brake on excessive glutamate signaling.

Pharmacological Strategies: Beyond Simple Agonism

The therapeutic potential of mGluRs is immense, but targeting them with traditional full agonists or antagonists often leads to unacceptable side effects due to the sheer volume of glutamate signaling in the brain. This challenge has driven a shift towards allosteric modulation.

Allosteric Modulators (PAMs and NAMs)

Allosteric modulators bind to a site distinct from the orthosteric (glutamate) binding site, often located within the transmembrane domain of the mGluR dimer. They do not activate the receptor themselves but modify its response to the endogenous ligand, glutamate.

- Positive Allosteric Modulators (PAMs): Bind to the receptor and increase the receptor's sensitivity or efficacy toward glutamate. They act like a 'volume knob,' turning up the signal only when the natural neurotransmitter is present. This is considered beneficial because it maintains the physiological control of the endogenous system, reducing the risk of widespread over-activation.
    - *Example:* An mGluR2 PAM enhances the inhibitory autoreceptor function only when glutamate is being released, helping to normalize excessive glutamate activity.
- Negative Allosteric Modulators (NAMs): Bind to the receptor and decrease its sensitivity or efficacy toward glutamate. They function as a 'volume knob' turning the signal down.

Clinical Relevance and Drug Development

The modulatory roles of mGluRs make them ideal targets for re-balancing dysfunctional neuronal circuits implicated in CNS disorders:

Target mGluR Group	Therapeutic Target (Primary Role)	Clinical Application (Therapeutic Goal)
Group I (mGluR5)	Excitatory / Plasticity Enhancement	Fragile X Syndrome (FXS): mGluR5 NAMs aim to reduce exaggerated downstream signaling pathways. Anxiety/Depression: mGluR5 NAMs are being explored to normalize hyper-excited states.

Group II (mGluR2/3)	Inhibitory Autoreceptor / Reduced Glutamate Release	Schizophrenia: mGluR2/3 PAMs aim to reduce excessive glutamatergic drive (hyperexcitation) thought to underlie some symptoms. Anxiety: mGluR2/3 agonists or PAMs reduce stress-induced glutamate release.
Group III (mGluR4)	Pre-synaptic Inhibition	Parkinson's Disease: mGluR4 PAMs can suppress hyperactivity in the basal ganglia, improving motor function.

The development of highly selective allosteric modulators for each mGluR subtype represents the cutting edge of psychopharmacology, offering the promise of treatments with unprecedented precision and fewer side effects compared to broad-acting drugs.

Summary

Metabotropic glutamate receptors stand as a testament to the sophistication of cellular signaling. As Family C GPCRs, their dimerization and unique VFT domain structure enable them to serve as fine-tuning mechanisms for the entire excitatory tone of the brain. The functional division into Group I (G_q-coupled excitation) and Groups II/III (G_i-coupled inhibition) provides a rich pharmacological landscape. Current drug development efforts, particularly those focused on Positive and Negative Allosteric Modulators, are capitalizing on this complexity. By offering a way to subtly adjust the activity of endogenous glutamate signaling rather than block it entirely, mGluR pharmacology holds the key to unlocking new treatments for a wide range of debilitating neurological and psychiatric conditions, promising a future of more targeted and nuanced therapeutic intervention.

CHAPTER 36

MUSCARINIC RECEPTORS

1. Introduction

Muscarinic receptors are a subtype of acetylcholine receptors that are G protein-coupled and play a central role in mediating parasympathetic nervous system activity. They are widely distributed in the central and peripheral nervous systems and influence a broad range of physiological functions including heart rate, glandular secretion, smooth muscle contraction, and cognitive function.

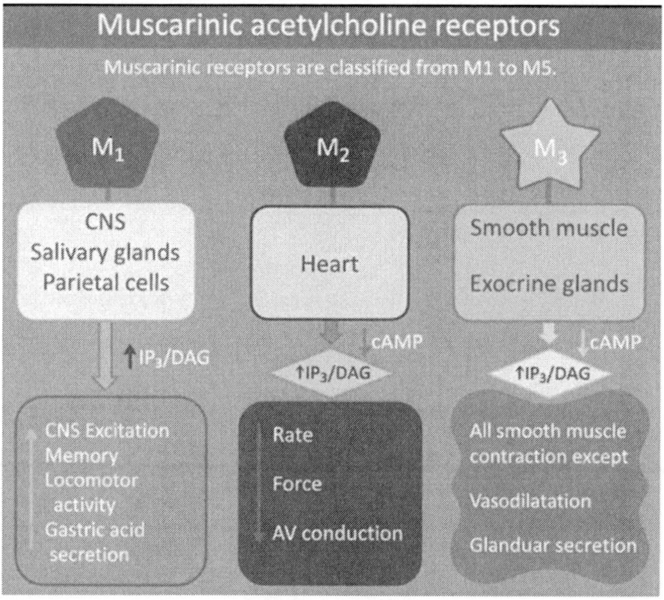

Fig 36.1 Muscarinic receptors, location and pharmacological actions.

Table 36.1 Muscarinic receptors classification and pharmacological actions.

Receptor Subtype	Second Messenger	Organ/Tissue	Response
M_1	IP_3/DAG ↑	Autonomic ganglion Brain (cerebral cortex) Gastric oxyntic cells	Slow EPSP Depolarization Increased gastric acid secretion via vagus nerve
M_2	cAMP ↓ and direct K^+ channel activation	Heart – atrium Sino-atrial node Prejunctional autonomic nerve endings Canine saphenous vein Ileum smooth muscle	Reduced twitch height and NA release Reduced rate (negative chronotropy) Reduced NA or ACh release Binding sites Predominant binding sites – uncertain function
M_3	IP_3/DAG ↑	Smooth muscle – gut Urinary bladder Trachea Iris circular muscle Blood vessels – endothelium Glands Oxyntic cells (gastric acid) Salivary glands Pancreatic β cells	Contraction Contraction Contraction Contraction Release of NO and vasodilatation Secretion Increased acid secretion Salivation Insulin release
M_4	cAMP ↓	Guinea-pig uterus Rabbit anococcygeus muscle Rabbit lung	Contraction NO-dependent relaxation Binding sites
M_5	IP_3/DAG ↑	Brain regions	Binding sites after all others occluded

2. Definition

Muscarinic receptors are G protein-coupled receptors (GPCRs) that respond to the endogenous neurotransmitter acetylcholine. Unlike nicotinic receptors which are ionotropic, muscarinic receptors mediate slower metabolic responses through second messenger systems.

3. Classification

Muscarinic receptors are classified into five subtypes based on pharmacological and molecular characteristics:

A. **M1 (Neural)**
   - Located in CNS, gastric parietal cells
   - Coupled to Gq → activates PLC → increases IP3 and DAG

B. **M2 (Cardiac)**
   - Found in heart, presynaptic neurons
   - Coupled to Gi → inhibits adenylate cyclase → decreases cAMP

C. **M3 (Glandular/Smooth Muscle)**
   - Present in exocrine glands, smooth muscle, endothelium
   - Coupled to Gq → activates PLC

D. **M4 (CNS, Striatum)**
   - Coupled to Gi/o

E. **M5 (CNS, Substantia Nigra)**
   - Coupled to Gq

4. Pharmacological Actions

Each muscarinic receptor subtype has distinct physiological effects:

I. **M1:** Enhances cognitive function and gastric acid secretion
II. **M2:** Slows heart rate and reduces atrial contractility
III. **M3:** Induces smooth muscle contraction (e.g., bronchi, bladder), promotes glandular secretion, causes vasodilation via NO release
IV. **M4 and M5:** Modulate dopamine release and motor function in the CNS

Muscarinic agonists mimic the action of acetylcholine, whereas antagonists block it. Common agonists include bethanechol and pilocarpine. Antagonists include atropine, ipratropium, and scopolamine.

5. Therapeutic Indications

Drugs targeting muscarinic receptors are used in various clinical settings:

I. **M1/M4:** Alzheimer's disease (e.g., xanomeline, experimental)
II. **M2:** Bradycardia management (atropine as antagonist)
III. **M3:**
   - Overactive bladder (e.g., oxybutynin, tolterodine)
   - Asthma and COPD (e.g., tiotropium, ipratropium)
   - Xerostomia (e.g., pilocarpine)
IV. **Preanesthetic medication:** Atropine reduces salivation and prevents vagal bradycardia
V. **Motion sickness:** Scopolamine (M1 antagonist)

6. Contraindications and Precautions

Use of muscarinic receptor drugs requires consideration of the following:

- **Glaucoma:** Anticholinergics may increase intraocular pressure
- **Prostatic Hypertrophy:** May worsen urinary retention
- **Myasthenia Gravis:** Anticholinergic drugs can worsen symptoms
- **Cardiac Disease:** Caution with M2 modulators due to risk of arrhythmias
- **Peptic Ulcers:** Cholinomimetics may increase gastric acid secretion

7. Summary

Muscarinic receptors are integral to parasympathetic nervous system function and are targeted for a wide range of therapeutic applications. The diversity of receptor subtypes allows for selective modulation, offering clinical utility in cardiology, pulmonology, neurology, and gastroenterology. Understanding their pharmacological profiles is essential for maximizing efficacy and minimizing adverse effects.

References

1. Eglen, R. M. (2006). Muscarinic receptor subtypes in neuronal and non-neuronal cholinergic function. *Autonomic & Autacoid Pharmacology*, 26(3), 219–233.

2. Wess, J. (2004). Muscarinic acetylcholine receptor knockout mice: novel phenotypes and clinical implications. *Annual Review of Pharmacology and Toxicology*, 44, 423–450.
3. Caulfield, M. P., & Birdsall, N. J. M. (1998). International Union of Pharmacology. XVII. Classification of muscarinic acetylcholine receptors. *Pharmacological Reviews*, 50(2), 279–290.
4. Duttaroy, A., &Gomeza, J. (2002). Role of M2 and M3 muscarinic receptors in the regulation of gastrointestinal motility. *Life Sciences*, 72(10), 1111–1117.
5. Felder, C. C. (1995). Muscarinic acetylcholine receptors: signal transduction through multiple second messenger systems. *Biochemical Pharmacology*, 49(3), 379–390.

CHAPTER 37

NICOTINIC ACETYLCHOLINE RECEPTORS

I. Definition

Nicotinic Acetylcholine Receptors (nAChRs) are a class of **ligand-gated ion channels (LGICs)**. These integral membrane proteins mediate fast synaptic transmission by converting the chemical signal of the neurotransmitter acetylcholine (ACh) into a rapid electrical signal [1, 5]. They are named "nicotinic" because they are selectively activated by the exogenous alkaloid nicotine [2].

- **Mechanism:** When two ACh molecules (or an agonist like nicotine) bind to the extracellular domain, the receptor undergoes a rapid conformational change, opening a central cation-permeable pore. The resulting influx of positive ions, primarily Na^+ and K^+ (and Ca^2+ in some subtypes), depolarizes the cell membrane, leading to an excitatory postsynaptic potential (EPSP) [2, 6].

II. Classification and Subunit Composition

nAChRs are pentameric (composed of five subunits) and belong to the Cys-loop family of receptors [1]. The composition determines their location, pharmacological profile, and ion permeability. There are 17 known mammalian subunits (\alpha 1-alpha 10, beta 1-beta 4, gamma, \delta, and \epsilon) [1].

Classification	Subunit Composition (Examples)	Location	Primary Function
Muscle Type	alpha 1_2 \beta 1 \delta \epsilon (Adult) or \alpha 1_2 \beta 1 \delta \gamma (Fetal/Embryonic)	**Neuromuscular Junction (NMJ)**	Mediates rapid, excitatory transmission leading to skeletal muscle contraction [2].

Ganglionic Type	$(\alpha 3)_2(\beta 4)_3$	**Autonomic Ganglia** (Sympathetic and Parasympathetic)	Transmits rapid excitatory impulses from pre-ganglionic neurons to post-ganglionic neurons [2].
Central Nervous System (CNS) Type	**Heteromeric:** $(\alpha 4)_2(\beta 2)_3$ or $(\alpha 4)_3(\beta 2)_2$ (Most common in brain) **Homomeric:** $(\alpha 7)_5$	**Brain** (e.g., VTA, Cortex, Hippocampus)	Modulates neurotransmitter release (presynaptic effect), memory, attention, and the reward pathway involved in addiction. $\alpha 7$ receptors are highly permeable to Ca^{2+} [2, 6].

III. Pharmacological Actions

Drugs targeting nAChRs are classified as agonists (stimulators) or antagonists (blockers).

A. Agonists (Activators)

- **Acetylcholine (ACh):** The endogenous neurotransmitter.
- **Nicotine:** Full agonist at most nAChR subtypes, particularly high affinity for $\alpha 4 \beta 2$ receptors (CNS type), driving its addictive properties [6].
- **Varenicline (Chantix):** A **partial agonist** selective for the $(\alpha 4)_2(\beta 2)_3$ subtype, used for smoking cessation [2].
- **Succinylcholine:** A **depolarizing blocker** that acts as an agonist but causes sustained depolarization, leading to channel desensitization and flaccid paralysis.

B. Antagonists (Blockers)

- **Non-depolarizing Neuromuscular Blockers:** (e.g., Rocuronium, Vecuronium, Tubocurarine) - Competitive antagonists at the muscle-type nAChR, preventing ACh binding and channel opening, resulting in skeletal muscle paralysis [2, 4].
- **Ganglionic Blockers:** (e.g., Hexamethonium, Mecamylamine) - Block the $\alpha 3 \beta 4$ (ganglionic) receptor type. Hexamethonium is a non-competitive antagonist

(channelblocker), while Mecamylamine is a competitive antagonist, though both have effects in the CNS [2].
- **\alpha-Bungarotoxin (\alpha-BTX):** A snake venom toxin that is a highly selective antagonist for the muscle-type and homomeric \alpha 7 receptors [2].

IV. Indications (Therapeutic Uses)

1. **Skeletal Muscle Paralysis:** Non-depolarizing neuromuscular blocking agents are critical in **general anesthesia** to facilitate endotracheal intubation and optimize surgical conditions (muscle relaxation) [2].
2. **Smoking Cessation: Varenicline** is used to reduce craving and withdrawal symptoms by partially stimulating the \alpha 4 \beta 2 receptors, while also preventing full activation by inhaled nicotine [2, 6].
3. **Neuropsychiatric Research:** Selective nAChR agonists and Positive Allosteric Modulators (PAMs), particularly those targeting the \alpha 7 subtype, are under investigation for treating cognitive deficits associated with **Alzheimer's disease** and **schizophrenia** [6].

V. Contraindications and Precautions

1. **Neuromuscular Blockers:**
   - **Absolute Contraindication:** Must **never** be administered without immediate access to mechanical ventilation due to paralysis of the diaphragm and respiratory muscles [2].
   - **Succinylcholine (Depolarizing Agent):** Contraindicated in patients with a history of Malignant Hyperthermia susceptibility, severe trauma/burns, or conditions causing pre-existing hyperkalemia, as it can worsen these states [2].
2. **Smoking Cessation Agents (Varenicline):**
   - Requires caution in patients with pre-existing psychiatric conditions or a history of suicidal ideation due to potential changes in mood and behavior, although the initial Black Box Warning has been revised [2].
3. **Ganglionic Blockers (e.g., Mecamylamine):**
   - Largely obsolete due to their non-specific effects on both sympathetic and parasympathetic systems, leading to severe side effects such as orthostatic hypotension and paralytic ileus.

References

1. IUPHAR/BPS Guide to PHARMACOLOGY. Nicotinic acetylcholine receptors (nACh). [Online resource for pharmacological data].
2. Katzung, B. G., Masters, S. B., & Trevor, A. J. *(e.g., Chapter 7, Cholinoceptor-Activating &Cholinoceptor-Blocking Drugs)*. **Basic and Clinical Pharmacology.** McGraw Hill Medical.
3. Rang, H. P., Dale, M. M., Ritter, J. M., Flower, R. J., & Henderson, G. *(e.g., Chapter 10, The Cholinergic System)*. **Rang and Dale's Pharmacology.** Elsevier.
4. Lüllmann, H., Mohr, K., & Wehling, M. *(e.g., Chapter 14, Cholinergic Agonists and Antagonists)*. **Color Atlas of Pharmacology.** Thieme.
5. Nicotinic acetylcholine receptor - Wikipedia. [Online encyclopedia article providing structural and pharmacological details].
6. Dani, J. A., & Bertrand, D. (2007). Nicotinic Acetylcholine Receptors and Nicotinic Cholinergic Mechanisms of the Central Nervous System. *Annual Review of Pharmacology and Toxicology*, 47, 699–729. [Review article detailing CNS function].

CHAPTER 38

PHARMACOLOGY OF THE N-METHYL-D-ASPARTATE (NMDA) RECEPTOR

The N-methyl-D-aspartate (NMDA) receptor is a highly complex, ionotropic glutamate receptor that mediates a slow, yet powerful, component of excitatory synaptic transmission in the central nervous system (CNS). It is crucial for synaptic plasticity, which is the cellular basis for learning and memory (Long-Term Potentiation, or LTP).

I. Structural Organization

The functional NMDA receptor is an obligate heterotetramer, typically composed of two obligatory glycine-binding GluN1 subunits and two glutamate-binding GluN2 subunits (GluN2A, 2B, 2C, or 2D). Combinations including GluN3 subunits (GluN3A or 3B) also exist and modulate function.

The receptor structure is organized into four main domains:

1. **Amino-Terminal Domain (ATD):** Located extracellularly, this domain is involved in allosteric modulation, particularly by zinc (Zn^2+) and certain antagonists (e.g., ifenprodil).
2. **Ligand-Binding Domain (LBD):** An extracellular "clamshell" structure where the primary agonists bind. The GluN1 subunit binds the co-agonist, typically **glycine** or D-**serine**, while the GluN2 subunit binds the primary neurotransmitter, **glutamate**.
3. **Transmembrane Domain (TMD):** Consists of three transmembrane helices (M1, M3, M4) and a re-entrant loop (M2) that forms the central ion channel pore. The M2 loop determines the channel's high Ca^2+ permeability.
4. **Carboxy-Terminal Domain (CTD):** An intracellular domain that anchors the receptor to the postsynaptic density, interacts with

numerous intracellular signaling proteins, and is a site for phosphorylation and trafficking regulation.

II. Unique Functional Properties: The Coincidence Detector

Unlike other ionotropic glutamate receptors (like AMPA receptors), NMDA receptors function as coincidence detectors, meaning channel opening requires two simultaneous conditions:

1. **Ligand Binding:** Simultaneous binding of glutamate to the GluN2 subunit and a co-agonist (typically glycine or D-serine) to the GluN1 subunit.
2. **Voltage-Dependent Block Removal:** The channel pore is blocked by an extracellular **magnesium ion (**Mg^{2+}**)** at resting membrane potential (≈ -70 mV). The cell must be substantially depolarized (e.g., by the activation of nearby AMPA receptors) to ≈ -30 mV to electrostatically repel the Mg^{2+} and unblock the channel.

Once activated and unblocked, the channel allows the influx of cations, predominantly Ca^{2+} and Na^{+}, and an efflux of K^{+}. The Ca^{2+} influx acts as a critical second messenger, triggering intracellular cascades essential for synaptic plasticity.

III. Pharmacological Targets and Agents

The NMDA receptor possesses multiple binding sites, which are targets for both endogenous modulators and therapeutic drugs.

Target Site Mechanism of Action Example Agents Clinical/Physiological Relevance

Glutamate Site (GluN2) Competitive Antagonism D-AP5 (D-APV), CPP Used extensively as research tools to block LTP.

Glycine/D-Serine Site (GluN1) Competitive Antagonism 7-Chlorokynurenate Co-agonist site modulation is a therapeutic focus for schizophrenia.

Pore/Channel Block (Within TMD) Uncompetitive Antagonism (Requires channel opening) Ketamine, Phencyclidine (PCP), Memantine

Dissociativeanesthetics (Ketamine), drugs of abuse (PCP), and Alzheimer's treatment (Memantine). Memantine is a low-affinity, use-dependent blocker that preferentially inhibits pathological tonic signaling (excitotoxicity).

Mg^2+ Site (Within TMD) Physiological Voltage-Dependent Block Magnesium Ions (Mg^2+) Essential for the receptor's function as a coincidence detector. Used clinically as an anti-convulsant (eclampsia).

Zn^2+ Site (Extracellular, GluN2A) Non-Competitive Allosteric Inhibition Zinc Ions (Zn^2+) Endogenous modulator; GluN2A-containing receptors are most sensitive.

ATD/Interface Sites Subunit-Selective Allosteric Modulation Ifenprodil, Ro25-6981 (Both are negative allosteric modulators for GluN2B-containing receptors) Allows for targeting specific receptor subtypes, which is critical for minimizing side effects.

IV. Pathophysiological and Therapeutic Importance

NMDA receptors are central to several neurological conditions:

- **Excitotoxicity:** Over-activation of NMDA receptors (e.g., during stroke or traumatic brain injury) leads to excessive Ca^2+ influx, which triggers cell death pathways. Antagonists like Memantine are designed to prevent this excessive, pathological signaling without blocking normal synaptic function.
- **Neurodegenerative Diseases:** Memantine is used to treat Alzheimer's disease by mitigating excitotoxicity associated with the disease.
- **Anesthesia and Depression:** Low-dose **Ketamine**, an NMDA channel blocker, is used as a fast-acting antidepressant and anesthetic. Its rapid antidepressant effect is thought to involve downstream effects following the transient blockade of NMDA receptors.
- **Schizophrenia:** Hypofunction of NMDA receptors is implicated in the cognitive and negative symptoms of schizophrenia. Therapies targeting the GluN1 co-agonist site (e.g., glycine transporter inhibitors or D-serine supplements) are being explored to boost NMDA function.

The diversity of NMDA receptor subunits (GluN2A-D) dictates their expression patterns, kinetics, and pharmacology, making them highly desirable targets for developing new, subtype-selective drugs with fewer side effects.

CHAPTER 39

NEUROMEDIN U RECEPTORS

1. Introduction

Neuromedin U (NMU) receptors are a class of G protein-coupled receptors (GPCRs) that mediate the biological actions of the neuropeptide neuromedin U, which is involved in regulating smooth muscle contraction, blood pressure, feeding behavior, stress response, and immune function. The discovery of these receptors has enhanced our understanding of neuropeptide signaling and its diverse physiological effects.

2. Definition

Neuromedin U receptors are GPCRs activated by the endogenous ligand neuromedin U, a neuropeptide originally isolated from porcine spinal cord and named for its ability to induce uterine smooth muscle contraction. There are two known subtypes in humans: NMUR1 and NMUR2.

3. Classification

Neuromedin U receptors belong to the Class A (rhodopsin-like) GPCR family and are classified into two major subtypes:

A. **NMUR1 (Neuromedin U Receptor 1):** Primarily expressed in peripheral tissues such as the gastrointestinal tract, pancreas, and adipose tissue and involved in peripheral regulation of metabolism and immune responses
B. **NMUR2 (Neuromedin U Receptor 2):** Predominantly expressed in the central nervous system, especially the hypothalamus and medulla and Regulates appetite, energy homeostasis, stress, and circadian rhythm

4. Pharmacological Actions

Neuromedin U receptors mediate a variety of biological actions by coupling primarily with Gq/11 proteins:

A. **NMUR1 Activation:** Stimulates phospholipase C → IP3 and DAG formation → intracellular Ca2+ release
   - o Promotes smooth muscle contraction, insulin secretion, and inflammatory cytokine production

B. **NMUR2 Activation:** Influences CNS functions such as food intake inhibition, stress response modulation, and regulation of body temperature and arousal

Emerging evidence suggests that NMU receptors also participate in immune cell signaling and neuroendocrine integration.

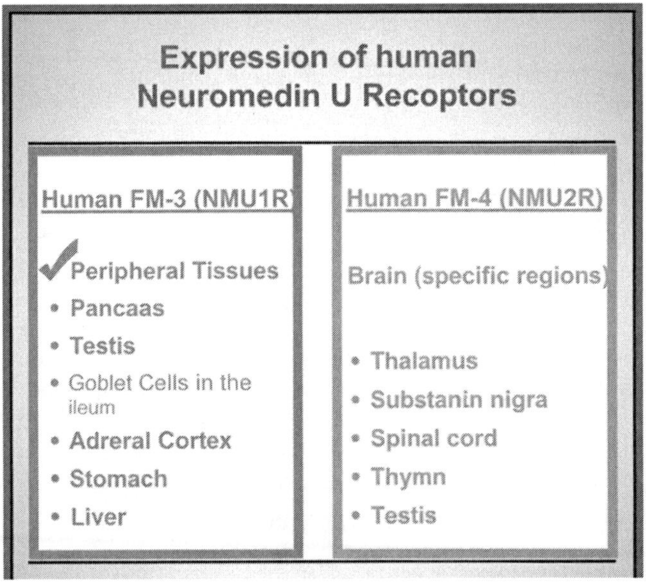

Fig. 39.1 Expression of human Neuromedin U receptors.

5. Therapeutic Indications

Though not yet targeted by approved clinical drugs, NMU receptors are being explored in preclinical and clinical research for:

I. **Obesity and Metabolic Disorders:** NMUR2 agonists may suppress appetite and increase energy expenditure
II. **Inflammatory Diseases:** NMUR1 modulation may help control cytokine production
III. **Stress-Related Disorders:** NMUR2 modulation could have anxiolytic or antidepressant effects
IV. **Gastrointestinal Disorders:** NMUR1 may regulate motility and secretion

6. Contraindications and Precautions

Due to the lack of approved drugs targeting NMU receptors, contraindications are theoretical and based on receptor distribution and function:

- **Cardiovascular Conditions:** NMU can increase blood pressure and heart rate
- **Autoimmune Disorders:** Excessive NMUR1 activation may exacerbate inflammation
- **Neuropsychiatric Disorders:** Central NMUR2 modulation may influence anxiety, sleep, or behavior
- **Pregnancy:** Effects on uterine contractility may contraindicate NMU analogs

7. Summary

Neuromedin U receptors are promising targets for multiple physiological systems including metabolism, immunity, and neuroendocrine function. Ongoing research into receptor-specific ligands may pave the way for new treatments in obesity, inflammatory diseases, and stress-related conditions.

References

1. Howard, A. D., Wang, R., Pong, S. S., et al. (2000). Identification of receptors for neuromedin U and its role in feeding. *Nature*, 406(6791), 70–74.
2. Brighton, P. J., Szekeres, P. G., & Willars, G. B. (2004). Neuromedin U and its receptors: structure, function, and physiological roles. *Pharmacology & Therapeutics*, 104(3), 233–266.

3. Takayama, K., Nagata, S., Tsubouchi, Y., et al. (2004). Molecular characterization and distribution of neuromedin U receptor subtype 2 in the rat brain. *Neuroscience Letters*, 370(2-3), 108–112.
4. Zhang, J. V., Ren, P. G., Avsian-Kretchmer, O., et al. (2006). Obestatin, a peptide encoded by the ghrelin gene, opposes ghrelin's effects on food intake. *Science*, 310(5750), 996–999.
5. Hedrick, J. A., Morse, K., Shan, L., et al. (2000). Identification of a human gastrointestinal tract and immune system receptor for the peptide neuromedin U. *Molecular Pharmacology*, 58(5), 870–875.

CHAPTER 40

NEUROPEPTIDE FF RECEPTORS: EMERGING ROLES IN PAIN MODULATION AND OPIOID SIGNALING

1. Introduction

Neuropeptide FF (NPFF) receptors are G protein-coupled receptors (GPCRs) that mediate the effects of neuropeptide FF, a member of the RFamide peptide family. These receptors are increasingly recognized for their involvement in pain modulation, opioid tolerance, cardiovascular regulation, and neuroendocrine signaling. Their distribution in both central and peripheral tissues underpins a diverse range of physiological and potential therapeutic functions.

2. Definition

NPFF receptors are GPCRs that respond to the endogenous ligands neuropeptide FF and neuropeptide AF. These peptides share a conserved Arg-Phe-NH2 (RFamide) motif at their C-terminus. Two subtypes of NPFF receptors have been identified: NPFFR1 and NPFFR2.

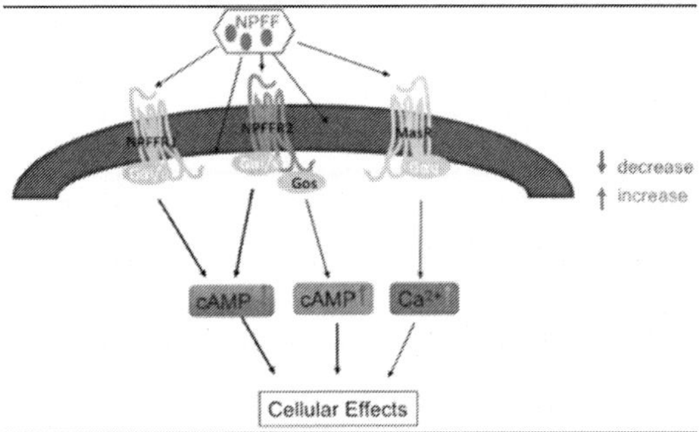

Fig. 35.1 Neuropeptide FF (NPFF) receptors pharmacological actions.

3. Classification

NPFF receptors belong to the Class A (rhodopsin-like) GPCR superfamily and are divided into:

A. **NPFFR1 (GPR147):**
   - Shows high affinity for neuropeptide AF
   - Predominantly expressed in the hypothalamus, spinal cord, and peripheral tissues

B. **NPFFR2 (GPR74):**
   - Preferentially activated by neuropeptide FF
   - Abundant in the brainstem, spinal cord, and sensory neurons

These receptors are distinct from other RFamide receptors such as prolactin-releasing peptide receptors or kisspeptin receptors.

4. Pharmacological Actions

NPFF receptors are known to couple primarily with Gi/o proteins, leading to:

- Inhibition of adenylate cyclase → decreased intracellular cAMP
- Activation of GIRK (G-protein-coupled inwardly rectifying potassium) channels
- Modulation of calcium channels and neurotransmitter release

Functional actions include:

1. **Pain Modulation:** NPFF acts as an anti-opioid peptide, attenuating opioid-induced analgesia and contributing to the development of opioid tolerance and hyperalgesia
2. **Endocrine Regulation:** Influences the hypothalamic-pituitary axis and stress responses
3. **Cardiovascular Control:** Modulates blood pressure and heart rate through central mechanisms
4. **Feeding and Metabolism:** Involvement in appetite suppression and energy homeostasis

5. Therapeutic Indications

Although no drugs targeting NPFF receptors are yet clinically approved, ongoing research supports potential applications in:

- **Opioid Tolerance Management:** Antagonists may enhance opioid analgesia and reduce tolerance
- **Chronic Pain Disorders:** Agonists or antagonists may offer new pathways for neuropathic and inflammatory pain treatment
- **Stress and Anxiety Disorders:** Central NPFFR2 signaling may modulate HPA axis activity
- **Cardiovascular Diseases:** Possible use in controlling neurogenic hypertension

6. Contraindications and Precautions

Potential contraindications for future NPFF receptor-based therapies would be theoretical at this stage but might include:

I. **Cardiovascular Conditions:** Due to effects on blood pressure and heart rate
II. **Mood Disorders:** Given their modulation of neuroendocrine systems, NPFF-targeting agents might impact mood or anxiety levels
III. **Drug Interactions:** With opioids, co-activation or blockade could alter analgesic efficacy and risk of dependence
IV. **Pregnancy:** Unknown effects on the fetal brain and neuroendocrine axis necessitate caution

7. Summary

NPFF receptors represent a promising area of neuropeptide pharmacology with significant implications for pain management, opioid use, and neuroendocrine regulation. Their unique ability to modulate opioid systems without direct opioid receptor engagement presents novel avenues for drug development, especially in combating opioid tolerance and dependence.

References

1. Panula, P., Kalso, E., Nieminen, L., et al. (1996). Neuropeptide FF, a mammalian neuropeptide with anti-opioid activity. *Nature*, 384(6604), 158–161.
2. Elhabazi, K., Humbert, J. P., Bertin, I., et al. (2006). Anti-opioid activities of RF-amide-related peptides: structure–activity relationship study. *Biochemical Pharmacology*, 72(9), 1097–1106.

3. Simonin, F., Schmitt, M., Laulin, J. P., et al. (2006). RF9, a selective antagonist of neuropeptide FF receptors, prevents morphine-induced tolerance associated with hyperalgesia. *PNAS*, 103(12), 4666–4671.
4. Hinuma, S., Habata, Y., Fujii, R., et al. (2000). New neuropeptides containing carboxy-terminal RFamide and their receptor in mammals. *Nature Cell Biology*, 2(10), 703–708.
5. Le Merrer, J., Becker, J. A. J., Befort, K., & Kieffer, B. L. (2009). Reward processing by the opioid system in the brain. *Physiological Reviews*, 89(4), 1379–1412.

CHAPTER 41

NEUROPEPTIDE S RECEPTORS: ROLE IN AROUSAL, ANXIETY, AND NEUROTRANSMISSION

1. Introduction

Neuropeptide S (NPS) and its cognate receptor (NPSR) have emerged as key modulators in the regulation of arousal, anxiety, locomotion, and neuroendocrine functions. Identified in 2004, the NPS-NPSR system represents a unique branch of neuropeptidergicsignaling in the central nervous system and holds promise for novel pharmacotherapeutic interventions, particularly in anxiety and sleep disorders.

2. Definition

The Neuropeptide S receptor (NPSR) is a G protein-coupled receptor (GPCR) that binds to the 20-amino acid neuropeptide S. Activation of NPSR by its ligand results in diverse physiological responses, primarily in the central nervous system.

3. Classification

NPSR belongs to the Class A (rhodopsin-like) family of GPCRs. It exists as a single known receptor subtype:

A. **NPSR1 (GPR154):** The only known functional receptor for NPS; expressed in the brainstem, amygdala, hypothalamus, and thalamus.

There are genetic polymorphisms (e.g., N107I) that modulate receptor responsiveness and have been linked to asthma, panic disorder, and other phenotypes.

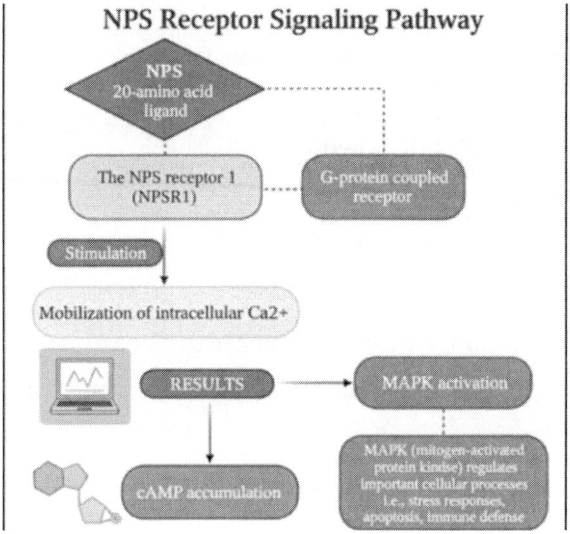

Fig. 41.1 Neuropeptide S Receptors signalling pathway.

4. Pharmacological Actions

Upon binding to NPS, NPSR couples primarily to the Gq and Gs proteins:

- **Gq Pathway:** Activates phospholipase C → increases IP3 and DAG → intracellular calcium release and PKC activation
- **Gs Pathway:** Stimulates adenylate cyclase → increases cAMP → activation of PKA

Key physiological effects include:

- **Stimulation of arousal and wakefulness**
- **Anxiolytic-like effects** (in rodent models)
- **Enhanced memory and learning**
- **Increased locomotor activity**
- **Suppression of appetite**

5. Therapeutic Indications

Though not yet approved for clinical use, the NPS-NPSR system is being explored for several potential applications:

I. **Anxiety Disorders:** Anxiolytic properties without sedation suggest utility in generalized anxiety or panic disorder
II. **Sleep Disorders:** Modulation of arousal without traditional sedative effects offers a new avenue in treating hypersomnia
III. **Asthma and Inflammation:** NPSR polymorphisms have been associated with airway hyperresponsiveness, suggesting anti-inflammatory potential
IV. **Cognitive Enhancement:** Potential in memory enhancement and neuroprotection

6. Contraindications and Precautions

While specific contraindications are theoretical at this stage, potential concerns include:

- ❖ **Hypertension and Tachycardia:** Due to arousal-promoting effects, may not be suitable for patients with cardiovascular disorders
- ❖ **Psychiatric Conditions:** Caution in bipolar disorder or schizophrenia due to central stimulatory properties
- ❖ **Pregnancy and Lactation:** Safety not established
- ❖ **Drug Interactions:** Possible synergistic effects with stimulants or anxiolytics

7. Summary

Neuropeptide S receptor signaling plays a pivotal role in regulating arousal and anxiety, offering a promising target for neuropsychiatric drug development. Future studies exploring biased agonism, receptor polymorphisms, and long-term effects will be crucial in translating preclinical findings into clinical therapies.

References

1. Xu, Y. L., Gall, C. M., Jackson, V. R., et al. (2004). A novel neuropeptide S stimulates arousal and anxiolytic-like effects in mice. *Journal of Neuroscience*, 24(18), 4473–4480.
2. Rizzi, A., Vergura, R., Marzola, G., et al. (2008). Neuropeptide S is a stimulatory anxiolytic agent: A behavioral and electrophysiological study in rats. *British Journal of Pharmacology*, 154(3), 471–479.

3. Leonard, S. K., & Ring, R. H. (2011). Immunohistochemical localization of the neuropeptide S receptor in the rat central nervous system. *Neuroscience*, 172, 153–163.
4. Reinscheid, R. K., Xu, Y. L., Okamura, N., et al. (2005). Pharmacological characterization of human and murine neuropeptide S receptors. *European Journal of Pharmacology*, 510(1–2), 9–16.
5. Okamura, N., Habay, S. A., Zeng, J., et al. (2008). Neuropeptide S receptor: A novel target for sleep and arousal regulation. *CNS & Neurological Disorders - Drug Targets*, 7(4), 348–360.

CHAPTER 42

NEUROPEPTIDE W RECEPTORS: PHYSIOLOGICAL FUNCTIONS AND PHARMACOLOGICAL SIGNIFICANCE

1. Introduction

Neuropeptide W (NPW) and its receptors are relatively recent discoveries in neuropeptide research. These receptors, part of the G protein-coupled receptor (GPCR) superfamily, are known for their roles in regulating stress responses, feeding behavior, endocrine secretion, and cardiovascular function. NPW functions alongside Neuropeptide B (NPB), and both peptides share receptors, thus often being studied in tandem.

2. Definition

Neuropeptide W receptors are GPCRs that specifically bind to NPW, modulating a range of neuroendocrine and autonomic responses. They are activated by endogenous peptides Neuropeptide W-23 and Neuropeptide W-30, named based on their amino acid lengths.

3. Classification

Neuropeptide W exerts its effects via two main receptors, both belonging to the Class A (rhodopsin-like) GPCR family:

A. **NPBWR1 (GPR7):** High affinity for both Neuropeptide W and Neuropeptide B. Widely expressed in the hypothalamus, amygdala, hippocampus, and other CNS regions.
B. **NPBWR2 (GPR8):** Present in humans but not rodents. Similar in function to NPBWR1 but with more restricted expression.

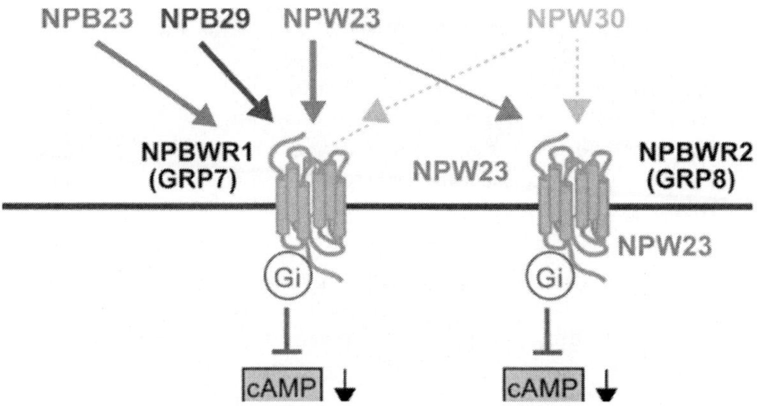

Fig 42.1 NPW receptors types and structure

4. Pharmacological Actions

Activation of NPW receptors leads to:

- **Gi/o protein coupling:** Inhibition of adenylate cyclase → reduction in cAMP levels → modulation of neurotransmitter release and hormone secretion
- **Gq/11 protein coupling (less common):** Activation of phospholipase C → increased IP3 and DAG → intracellular calcium mobilization

Physiological effects include:

- Regulation of feeding and energy homeostasis
- Modulation of stress responses (hypothalamic-pituitary-adrenal axis)
- Influence on neuroendocrine functions, particularly in corticotropin-releasing hormone secretion
- Control of cardiovascular parameters such as blood pressure and heart rate
- Effects on pain perception and emotion regulation

5. Therapeutic Indications

While clinical use of NPW receptor-targeting drugs is still under investigation, potential indications include:

I. **Obesity and Metabolic Disorders:** Due to their anorexigenic effects and role in energy balance
II. **Anxiety and Stress-Related Disorders:** Given their regulation of the HPA axis and expression in limbic regions
III. **Hypertension:** Owing to modulatory effects on blood pressure
IV. **Neuroendocrine Tumors or Dysfunctions:** Via their regulatory role in hormone secretion

6. Contraindications and Precautions

As receptor-targeting drugs are under development, theoretical contraindications include:

- **Hypotension:** In patients prone to low blood pressure, as receptor activation may influence vascular tone
- **Psychiatric Conditions:** Caution due to potential modulation of mood and behavior
- **Endocrine Disorders:** Because of influence on hypothalamic and pituitary hormones
- **Pregnancy and Lactation:** Safety profile not yet established

7. Summary

Neuropeptide W receptors represent an intriguing class of GPCRs with broad physiological and pharmacological relevance. Their dual role in metabolic and neuroendocrine regulation makes them promising targets for treating obesity, stress disorders, and cardiovascular conditions. Future therapeutic development will benefit from advances in selective receptor agonists/antagonists and further understanding of receptor signaling pathways.

References

1. Tanaka, M., Shintani, Y., Fukuhara, S., et al. (2003). Neuropeptide W participates in the hypothalamic regulation of feeding behavior. *Nature*, 422(6928), 512–518.
2. Brezillon, S., Lannoy, V., Franssen, J. D., et al. (2003). Identification of natural ligands for the orphan G protein-coupled receptors GPR7 and GPR8. *Journal of Biological Chemistry*, 278(4), 776–783.
3. Lee, D. K., Nguyen, T., Porter, C. A., et al. (1999). Characterization of novel receptors GPR7 and GPR8 as endogenous receptors for

neuropeptides B and W. *Journal of Biological Chemistry*, 274(41), 31459–31464.

4. Fukusumi, S., Fujii, R., Hinuma, S. (2006). Recent progress in neuropeptide research: Focus on neuropeptide B and neuropeptide W. *Pharmacology & Therapeutics*, 112(3), 471–487.
5. Mondal, M. S., Yamaguchi, H., Date, Y., et al. (2003). Neuropeptide W decreases food intake through hypothalamic activation in rats. *Biochemical and Biophysical Research Communications*, 311(4), 954–958.

CHAPTER 43

NEUROPEPTIDE Y RECEPTORS: NEUROPHYSIOLOGICAL ROLES AND THERAPEUTIC RELEVANCE

1. Introduction

Neuropeptide Y (NPY) is a 36-amino acid peptide that is one of the most abundant neuropeptides in the mammalian brain. It plays a pivotal role in regulating various physiological functions including appetite, circadian rhythm, anxiety, cardiovascular function, and energy homeostasis. NPY mediates its effects through a family of G protein-coupled receptors (GPCRs), making them critical targets in pharmacology.

2. Definition

Neuropeptide Y receptors are GPCRs that bind NPY and related peptides such as peptide YY (PYY) and pancreatic polypeptide (PP). These receptors mediate their actions by coupling primarily to Gi/o proteins, thereby inhibiting adenylate cyclase and modulating intracellular signaling cascades.

3. Classification

The NPY receptor family includes multiple subtypes with distinct distribution and physiological roles:

A. **Y1 receptor:** Widely expressed in the brain and peripheral tissues; involved in feeding behavior and vasoconstriction.
B. **Y2 receptor:** Functions as an autoreceptor on NPY neurons; modulates neurotransmitter release.
C. **Y4 receptor:** Preferentially binds pancreatic polypeptide; involved in gastrointestinal function.

D. **Y5 receptor:** Implicated in the regulation of food intake and obesity.
E. **Y6 receptor:** Present in some species; its function remains unclear in humans due to a nonfunctional pseudogene.

4. Pharmacological Actions

NPY receptors, through Gi/o protein coupling, typically:

- Inhibit adenylate cyclase → reduce cAMP levels
- Modulate ion channel activity → affect neuronal excitability
- Influence gene expression and neuropeptide release

Functional outcomes:

- **Appetite stimulation (Y1, Y5):** Increases food intake
- **Inhibition of neurotransmitter release (Y2):** Reduces presynaptic release of NPY and other transmitters
- **Vasoconstriction (Y1):** Raises blood pressure
- **Stress response and anxiolysis:** Involvement in limbic system regulation

5. Therapeutic Indications

NPY receptor modulators have potential in the treatment of:

- **Obesity and Eating Disorders:** Y1 and Y5 receptor antagonists to reduce appetite
- **Anxiety and Depression:** Y1 and Y2 modulation to affect stress response
- **Cardiovascular Disorders:** Y1 receptor antagonists may reduce hypertension
- **Epilepsy:** Y2 receptor agonists have shown anticonvulsant properties in preclinical models

6. Contraindications and Precautions

Therapeutic manipulation of NPY receptors must be approached cautiously due to their wide physiological impact:

- **Cardiovascular Risk:** Y1 antagonism may reduce vasoconstriction but affect blood pressure control
- **Metabolic Disruption:** Prolonged blockade of Y5 may impair energy balance
- **Neuropsychiatric Effects:** Modulation may alter mood, stress resilience, or behavior
- **Pregnancy and Lactation:** Effects on fetal and neonatal development are not well studied

7. Summary

Neuropeptide Y receptors represent a complex, multifaceted system with profound implications in appetite regulation, stress, cardiovascular function, and neurological disorders. Continued development of subtype-selective ligands offers promise for treating obesity, anxiety, and hypertension, though clinical translation requires careful evaluation of systemic effects.

References

1. Michel, M. C., Beck-Sickinger, A., Cox, H., et al. (1998). XVI. International Union of Pharmacology recommendations for the nomenclature of neuropeptide Y, peptide YY, and pancreatic polypeptide receptors. *Pharmacological Reviews*, 50(1), 143–150.
2. Pedrazzini, T., Pralong, F., &Grouzmann, E. (2003). Neuropeptide Y: the universal soldier. *Cellular and Molecular Life Sciences*, 60(2), 350–377.
3. Naveilhan, P., Hassani, H., Canals, J. M., et al. (2001). Normal feeding behavior, body weight and leptin response require the neuropeptide Y Y2 receptor. *Nature Medicine*, 7(10), 1053–1059.
4. Kuo, L. E., Kitlinska, J. B., & Tilan, J. U. (2007). Neuropeptide Y acts directly in the periphery on fat tissue and mediates stress-induced obesity and metabolic syndrome. *Nature Medicine*, 13(7), 803–811.
5. Zambello, E., Cheung, L., & Buckley, T. L. (2022). Y-receptor signaling in the central nervous system: Current therapeutic developments. *Frontiers in Neuroscience*, 16, 854739.

CHAPTER 44

NEUROTENSIN RECEPTORS: MOLECULAR PHARMACOLOGY AND CLINICAL POTENTIAL

1. Introduction

Neurotensin is a 13-amino acid neuropeptide that functions as both a neurotransmitter and a hormone. It modulates a variety of central and peripheral physiological processes including nociception, temperature regulation, dopaminergic neurotransmission, and gastrointestinal activity. Neurotensin receptors mediate these effects and are emerging as targets in neuropsychiatric and gastrointestinal disorders.

2. Definition

Neurotensin receptors are a class of G protein-coupled receptors (GPCRs) that bind neurotensin to initiate downstream signaling cascades. These receptors are found in both the central nervous system (CNS) and peripheral tissues.

3. Classification

There are three known subtypes of neurotensin receptors:

A. **NTS1 (Neurotensin receptor type 1):** High-affinity receptor that couples with Gq/11 proteins, leading to activation of phospholipase C and calcium signaling.
B. **NTS2 (Neurotensin receptor type 2):** Lower affinity; signaling pathways are less well defined, but may involve Gi/o and ion channel modulation.
C. **NTS3 (Sortilin):** Not a classical GPCR; involved in intracellular trafficking and signaling pathways.

4. Pharmacological Actions

Neurotensin receptor activation influences a broad range of physiological processes:

A. **NTS1:**
   - ❖ Stimulates phospholipase C → IP3 and DAG formation → increases intracellular Ca^{2+}
   - ❖ Modulates dopaminergic pathways in the CNS
   - ❖ Induces hypothermia, analgesia, and modulation of locomotion

B. **NTS2:** Involved in analgesia and modulation of anxiety

C. **NTS3 (Sortilin):**
   - ❖ Regulates neurotensin internalization and trafficking
   - ❖ May participate in apoptotic pathways and lipid metabolism

5. Therapeutic Indications

Therapeutic interest in neurotensin receptors has increased due to their roles in several pathophysiological conditions:

I. **Schizophrenia and Psychosis:** NTS1 agonists enhance dopaminergic modulation and show antipsychotic-like effects

II. **Pain Management:** NTS2-selective agonists offer analgesic effects without opioids

III. **Cancer:** Overexpression of NTS1 in certain cancers (e.g., pancreatic, prostate, and colorectal) suggests potential for targeted therapies

IV. **Gastrointestinal Disorders:** Modulation of GI motility and secretion via NTS1 receptors

6. Contraindications and Precautions

While preclinical research is promising, potential therapeutic use of neurotensin receptor modulators must consider the following:

- ❖ **Hypotension and Hypothermia:** NTS1 agonists may lower blood pressure and body temperature
- ❖ **Neurological Effects:** Dysregulation of dopaminergic activity can lead to motor side effects or psychiatric symptoms
- ❖ **Oncogenic Risk:** Overactivation of NTS1 could promote tumor growth in susceptible tissues

- **Drug Interactions:** Caution when used with other CNS-acting agents due to potential synergistic effects

7. Summary

Neurotensin receptors are involved in numerous physiological and pathological processes, making them attractive targets for novel therapies in neuropsychiatric, oncological, and pain-related conditions. Further research is needed to develop selective modulators and assess long-term safety profiles.

References

1. Vincent, J. P., Mazella, J., &Kitabgi, P. (1999). Neurotensin and neurotensin receptors. *Trends in Pharmacological Sciences*, 20(7), 302–309.
2. Mustain, W. C., Rychahou, P. G., & Evers, B. M. (2011). The role of neurotensin in physiologic and pathologic processes. *Current Opinion in Endocrinology, Diabetes and Obesity*, 18(1), 75–82.
3. Binder, E. B., Kinkead, B., Owens, M. J., & Nemeroff, C. B. (2001). Neurotensin and dopamine interactions. *Pharmacological Reviews*, 53(4), 453–486.
4. Boules, M., Fredrickson, P., Myers, R., & Richelson, E. (2006). Neurotensin receptor agonists: a promising class of neurotherapeutics. *Annals of the New York Academy of Sciences*, 1070, 543–549.
5. Dupouy, S., Mourra, N., Doan, V. K., et al. (2009). The neurotensin receptor-1 pathway contributes to human ductal breast cancer progression. *PLoS One*, 4(1), e4223.

CHAPTER 45

OPIOID RECEPTORS: CLASSIFICATION, MECHANISMS, AND THERAPEUTIC APPLICATIONS

1. Introduction

Opioid receptors are a group of G protein-coupled receptors (GPCRs) that mediate the effects of endogenous opioid peptides (e.g., endorphins, enkephalins, dynorphins) and exogenous opioid drugs (e.g., morphine, fentanyl). They play a central role in pain modulation, reward, stress response, and autonomic regulation.

2. Definition

Opioid receptors are GPCRs that respond to opioid ligands to initiate intracellular signaling cascades, primarily through inhibition of adenylyl cyclase, activation of potassium channels, and inhibition of calcium channels, resulting in decreased neuronal excitability.

3. Classification

There are three primary opioid receptor subtypes:

A. **Mu (μ) Opioid Receptors (MOR):**
   - ❖ High affinity for morphine and β-endorphins
   - ❖ Responsible for analgesia, euphoria, respiratory depression, and physical dependence

B. **Delta (δ) Opioid Receptors (DOR):**
   - ❖ Bind enkephalins preferentially
   - ❖ Involved in analgesia, mood regulation, and neuroprotection

C. **Kappa (κ) Opioid Receptors (KOR):**
   - ❖ Bind dynorphins
   - ❖ Mediate analgesia, diuresis, and dysphoria

D. **Nociceptin/Orphanin FQ Receptor (NOP or ORL1):**
   - Structurally similar but pharmacologically distinct from classical opioid receptors
   - Involved in pain, mood, and drug reward regulation

4. Pharmacological Actions

Opioid receptors modulate neurotransmitter release and neural excitability. Major effects include:

- **Analgesia:** Inhibition of pain pathways in the spinal cord and brain
- **Euphoria and Reward:** Activation of mesolimbic dopaminergic pathways (primarily MOR)
- **Respiratory Depression:** Inhibition of brainstem respiratory centers
- **Sedation:** Reduction in CNS excitability
- **Gastrointestinal Effects:** Inhibition of gastrointestinal motility leading to constipation

5. Therapeutic Indications

Opioid receptor agonists and antagonists are used in a variety of clinical settings:

I. **Pain Management:**
   - Morphine, fentanyl, oxycodone (MOR agonists)
   - Used in acute and chronic pain, cancer pain, postoperative pain

II. **Anesthesia Adjuncts:**
   - Remifentanil and sufentanil

III. **Opioid Dependence:**
   - Methadone and buprenorphine (partial MOR agonists)
   - Naltrexone and naloxone (MOR antagonists)

IV. **Diarrhea Treatment:**
   - Loperamide (peripherally acting MOR agonist)

V. **Cough Suppression:**
   - Codeine and dextromethorphan

6. Contraindications and Precautions

Use of opioid drugs must be closely monitored due to serious risks:

- **Respiratory Depression:** Major cause of opioid-related mortality, especially in overdose
- **Addiction and Dependence:** Long-term use leads to tolerance and physical/psychological dependence
- **CNS Depression:** Potentiated by other sedatives, alcohol, or benzodiazepines
- **Pregnancy and Lactation:** Risk of neonatal withdrawal syndrome and respiratory depression in infants
- **Contraindicated Conditions:**
    - Head injury (risk of increased intracranial pressure)
    - Severe asthma or respiratory insufficiency

Clinical Importance

Mu-opioid receptor — Naloxone reversal of opioid overdose

Vignette idea: Emergency reversal of respiratory depression in intravenous opioid overdose using naloxone; discuss competitive antagonism at μ-opioid receptors, dosing considerations, and risk of withdrawal.

Reference: Jordan MR, et al. Naloxone. StatPearls. 2024. NCBI+1

CHAPTER 46

OREXIN RECEPTORS: CLASSIFICATION, MECHANISMS, AND CLINICAL APPLICATIONS

1. Introduction

Orexin receptors are G protein-coupled receptors (GPCRs) that bind neuropeptides orexin A and orexin B (also known as hypocretins). Discovered in the late 1990s, these receptors are integral to the regulation of sleep-wake cycles, arousal, energy homeostasis, and appetite. They are primarily expressed in the central nervous system, especially in the hypothalamus, and have gained therapeutic significance in sleep disorders and metabolic regulation.

2. Definition

Orexin receptors are GPCRs activated by the endogenous ligands orexin A and B, which modulate various neurophysiological processes including wakefulness, feeding behavior, and reward systems. They are coupled primarily to Gq proteins but can also interact with other G protein subtypes depending on the cellular context.

3. Classification

There are two main subtypes of orexin receptors:

A. **Orexin Receptor Type 1 (OX1R):**
   - ❖ Has a higher affinity for orexin A than orexin B
   - ❖ Predominantly linked to arousal and reward-seeking behavior

B. **Orexin Receptor Type 2 (OX2R):**
   - ❖ Binds both orexin A and B with similar affinity
   - ❖ Plays a major role in regulating sleep-wake cycles and energy metabolism

4. Pharmacological Actions

Activation of orexin receptors leads to increased intracellular calcium levels and activation of downstream signaling pathways that enhance neuronal excitability and neurotransmitter release. Key actions include:

- ❖ **Promotion of Wakefulness:** Orexin neurons stimulate monoaminergic and cholinergic systems
- ❖ **Stimulation of Feeding:** Activation of hypothalamic pathways involved in hunger signaling
- ❖ **Enhancement of Reward Responses:** Interaction with dopaminergic neurons in the ventral tegmental area (VTA)
- ❖ **Regulation of Energy Balance:** Influence on thermogenesis and locomotor activity

5. Therapeutic Indications

Pharmacological modulation of orexin receptors has emerged as a promising therapeutic strategy:

- ❖ **Insomnia:** Dual orexin receptor antagonists (DORAs) like suvorexant and lemborexant promote sleep by inhibiting both OX1R and OX2R
- ❖ **Narcolepsy:** Orexin receptor agonists (under development) aim to restore wakefulness in narcoleptic patients
- ❖ **Addiction and Reward Disorders:** Potential targets for reducing drug-seeking behaviors
- ❖ **Obesity and Metabolic Disorders:** Experimental role in modulating appetite and energy expenditure

6. Contraindications and Precautions

Use of orexin receptor modulators should be approached with caution in specific clinical contexts:

- **Daytime Somnolence:** Antagonists may cause next-day drowsiness and impaired cognitive function
- **Depression and Suicidality:** Some DORAs carry warnings due to reported psychiatric side effects
- **Liver Impairment:** Metabolism of drugs like suvorexant involves hepatic pathways, requiring dose adjustment

- **Concomitant Use with CNS Depressants:** Additive effects may increase the risk of respiratory depression
- **Pregnancy and Lactation:** Limited safety data available; use only if benefits outweigh risks

7. Summary

Orexin receptors are vital to the maintenance of wakefulness and energy balance, and represent a novel class of drug targets in sleep and metabolic disorders. Advances in the development of receptor-selective antagonists and agonists hold great promise for clinical application in neuropsychiatric and metabolic conditions.

References

1. Sakurai, T. (2007). The neural circuit of orexin (hypocretin): maintaining sleep and wakefulness. *Nature Reviews Neuroscience*, 8(3), 171–181.
2. Winrow, C. J., & Renger, J. J. (2014). Discovery and development of orexin receptor antagonists as therapeutics for insomnia. *British Journal of Pharmacology*, 171(2), 283–293.
3. Dauvilliers, Y., Bassetti, C., Lammers, G. J., et al. (2020). Pitolisant versus placebo in patients with narcolepsy: A double-blind, randomized trial. *Lancet Neurology*, 19(11), 902–913.
4. Mahoney, C. E., Cogswell, A., Koralnik, I. J., & Scammell, T. E. (2019). The neurobiological basis of narcolepsy. *Nature Reviews Neuroscience*, 20(2), 83–93.
5. Brisbare-Roch, C., Dingemanse, J., Koberstein, R., et al. (2007). Promotion of sleep by targeting the orexin system in rats, dogs and humans. *Nature Medicine*, 13(2), 150–155.

CHAPTER 47

P2Y RECEPTORS: STRUCTURE, FUNCTION, AND THERAPEUTIC POTENTIAL

1. Introduction

P2Y receptors are a subfamily of purinergic G protein-coupled receptors (GPCRs) that respond to extracellular nucleotides such as ATP, ADP, UTP, and UDP. These receptors play essential roles in various physiological processes, including platelet aggregation, inflammation, vascular tone regulation, and neurotransmission.

2. Definition

P2Y receptors are metabotropic purinergic receptors that are activated by nucleotides and are involved in signal transduction via G proteins. Unlike P2X receptors, which are ligand-gated ion channels, P2Y receptors modulate cellular responses through second messengers such as cAMP and intracellular calcium.

3. Classification

The human P2Y receptor family includes eight well-characterized subtypes, divided based on their ligand specificity and G protein coupling:

A. **P2Y1**
B. **P2Y2**
C. **P2Y4**
D. **P2Y6**
E. **P2Y11**
F. **P2Y12**
G. **P2Y13**
H. **P2Y14**

Ligand Specificity:

- **ATP/ADP-sensitive:** P2Y1, P2Y11, P2Y12, P2Y13
- **UTP/UDP-sensitive:** P2Y2, P2Y4, P2Y6, P2Y14

G Protein Coupling:

- **Gq/11-coupled:** P2Y1, P2Y2, P2Y4, P2Y6, P2Y11 (stimulate PLC → IP3/DAG pathway → Ca2+ signaling)
- **Gi/o-coupled:** P2Y12, P2Y13, P2Y14 (inhibit adenylate cyclase → reduce cAMP levels)

4. Pharmacological Actions

P2Y receptors mediate various cellular responses depending on their subtype and tissue distribution:

I. **Platelet Aggregation:** P2Y1 and P2Y12 activation promotes ADP-induced platelet activation
II. **Immune Modulation:** P2Y6 and P2Y14 participate in cytokine release and chemotaxis
III. **Vasodilation/Vasoconstriction:** P2Y2 and P2Y4 are involved in endothelial-mediated vascular responses
IV. **Neurotransmission and Neuroprotection:** P2Y receptors modulate synaptic transmission and glial cell activity

5. Therapeutic Indications

Several drugs targeting P2Y receptors have been developed, especially in cardiovascular and inflammatory disorders:

- **Thrombosis and Cardiovascular Disease:** P2Y12 antagonists (e.g., clopidogrel, prasugrel, ticagrelor) prevent platelet aggregation
- **Cystic Fibrosis:** P2Y2 agonists are explored for improving airway hydration
- **Inflammatory Diseases:** P2Y6 and P2Y14 modulators are under investigation for immune-related conditions
- **Neurological Disorders:** Potential roles in neurodegenerative disease management are being studied

6. Contraindications and Precautions

Caution must be exercised with drugs targeting P2Y receptors due to potential side effects:

- **Bleeding Risk:** P2Y12 inhibitors increase bleeding tendency and are contraindicated in active bleeding conditions
- **Drug Resistance and Metabolism:** Genetic polymorphisms (e.g., CYP2C19 for clopidogrel) can affect drug efficacy
- **Hepatic and Renal Impairment:** Dose adjustments may be required depending on the receptor-targeting drug's clearance
- **Concomitant Anticoagulants:** Risk of additive anticoagulant effect and bleeding

7. Summary

P2Y receptors are critical regulators of purinergic signaling in the cardiovascular, immune, and nervous systems. Their pharmacological modulation offers valuable therapeutic avenues, particularly in antiplatelet therapy. Continued research on receptor subtype specificity and downstream signaling may yield novel treatments for a broad range of diseases.

References

1. Abbracchio, M. P., Burnstock, G., Boeynaems, J. M., et al. (2006). International Union of Pharmacology LVIII: Update on the P2Y G protein-coupled nucleotide receptors: From molecular mechanisms and pathophysiology to therapy. *Pharmacological Reviews*, 58(3), 281–341.
2. Burnstock, G., & Knight, G. E. (2004). Cellular distribution and functions of P2 receptor subtypes in different systems. *International Review of Cytology*, 240, 31–304.
3. Jacobson, K. A., &Boeynaems, J. M. (2010). P2Y nucleotide receptors: promise of therapeutic applications. *Drug Discovery Today*, 15(13-14), 570–578.
4. Hollopeter, G., Jantzen, H. M., Vincent, D., et al. (2001). Identification of the platelet ADP receptor targeted by antithrombotic drugs. *Nature*, 409(6817), 202–207.
5. von Kügelgen, I. (2006). Pharmacological profiles of cloned mammalian P2Y-receptor subtypes. *Pharmacology & Therapeutics*, 110(3), 415–432.

CHAPTER 48

PARATHYROID HORMONE RECEPTORS: STRUCTURE, SIGNALING, AND CLINICAL APPLICATIONS

1. Introduction

Parathyroid hormone receptors (PTHRs) are critical components of calcium and phosphate homeostasis, bone remodeling, and renal function. These receptors, particularly activated by parathyroid hormone (PTH) and parathyroid hormone-related peptide (PTHrP), are important targets for therapies in osteoporosis and hypoparathyroidism.

2. Definition

Parathyroid hormone receptors are G protein-coupled receptors (GPCRs) that bind PTH and PTHrP. They mediate the biological effects of these hormones by activating multiple intracellular signaling cascades primarily through G proteins.

3. Classification

There are two major subtypes of PTH receptors:

A. **PTH1 Receptor (PTH1R):**
   - ❖ Predominantly expressed in bone and kidney
   - ❖ Binds both PTH and PTHrP with high affinity

B. **PTH2 Receptor (PTH2R):**
   - ❖ Primarily expressed in the central nervous system, pancreas, and placenta
   - ❖ Selectively binds PTH but not PTHrP

4. Pharmacological Actions

PTH receptors mediate their effects via G protein signaling:

- **Gs protein pathway:** Activates adenylate cyclase → increases cAMP → activates PKA → regulates gene transcription (e.g., RANKL, osteocalcin)
- **Gq/11 protein pathway:** Activates phospholipase C → increases IP3 and DAG → elevates intracellular Ca^{2+} → activates PKC

These pathways result in:

- Bone resorption or formation (depending on exposure duration)
- Renal reabsorption of calcium and excretion of phosphate
- Modulation of vitamin D metabolism

5. Therapeutic Indications

Drugs targeting PTH receptors are employed in treating various metabolic bone diseases:

I. **Osteoporosis:** Teriparatide (recombinant PTH 1-34) is an anabolic agent stimulating bone formation via PTH1R
II. **Hypoparathyroidism:** Recombinant full-length PTH (e.g., Natpara) restores calcium balance
III. **Fracture Healing:** PTHanalogs are investigated for accelerating fracture repair

6. Contraindications and Precautions

Use of PTH receptor agonists requires careful risk assessment:

- **Osteosarcoma Risk:** Long-term use is associated with increased osteosarcoma risk in rodent studies; limited duration of therapy recommended
- **Hypercalcemia:** Avoid in patients with pre-existing hypercalcemia
- **Paget's Disease or Skeletal Metastases:** Contraindicated due to potential for abnormal bone turnover
- **Renal Impairment:** Risk of altered calcium and phosphate handling
- **Pregnancy and Lactation:** Limited safety data; use only if benefits outweigh risks

7. Summary

Parathyroid hormone receptors are integral to skeletal and renal physiology and are prime targets in treating bone disorders. Advances in receptor biology and selective analog development have significantly enhanced therapeutic outcomes while minimizing adverse effects. Continued research may yield next-generation PTH receptor modulators with improved safety profiles.

References

1. Gardella, T. J., &Vilardaga, J. P. (2015). International Union of Basic and Clinical Pharmacology. XCIII. The parathyroid hormone receptors—family B G protein-coupled receptors. *Pharmacological Reviews*, 67(2), 310–337.
2. Jüppner, H. (2000). Phosphate and FGF-23. *Kidney International*, 57(Suppl 77), S8–S12.
3. Potts, J. T., & Gardella, T. J. (2007). Progress, paradox, and potential: Parathyroid hormone research over five decades. *Journal of Bone and Mineral Research*, 22(12), 1835–1841.
4. Datta, N. S., & Abou-Samra, A. B. (2009). PTH and PTHrPsignaling in osteoblasts. *Cellular Signalling*, 21(8), 1245–1254.
5. Neer, R. M., Arnaud, C. D., Zanchetta, J. R., et al. (2001). Effect of parathyroid hormone (1-34) on fractures and bone mineral density in postmenopausal women with osteoporosis. *New England Journal of Medicine*, 344(19), 1434–1441.

CHAPTER 49

PLATELET RECEPTORS: STRUCTURE, FUNCTION, AND CLINICAL IMPLICATIONS

1. Introduction

Platelet receptors are membrane-bound proteins expressed on the surface of platelets that mediate platelet adhesion, activation, aggregation, and signal transduction during hemostasis and thrombosis. Understanding platelet receptor biology is crucial for managing thrombotic disorders and developing antiplatelet therapies.

2. Definition

Platelet receptors are specific cell surface receptors that recognize and bind to soluble or immobilized ligands such as collagen, thrombin, ADP, thromboxane A2, and fibrinogen. These receptors initiate intracellular signaling cascades leading to platelet activation and aggregation.

3. Classification of Platelet Receptors

Platelet receptors are classified based on their ligands and signaling pathways:

A. **Integrin Receptors**
   - **αIIbβ3 (GPIIb/IIIa):** Binds fibrinogen and von Willebrand factor (vWF)
   - **α2β1:** Binds collagen

B. **G Protein-Coupled Receptors (GPCRs)**
   - **P2Y12 and P2Y1:** ADP receptors
   - **TP (Thromboxane receptor):** Binds thromboxane A2
   - **PAR-1 and PAR-4:** Protease-activated receptors, activated by thrombin

C. **Glycoprotein Receptors**
   - **GPIb-IX-V complex:** Binds vWF
   - **GPVI:** Binds collagen, major collagen receptor for activation

D. **Other Receptors**
   - **CLEC-2:** Activated by podoplanin
   - **FcγRIIA:** Low-affinity IgG receptor, mediates immune-related platelet activation

4. Pharmacological Actions

Platelet receptors initiate multiple intracellular signaling cascades upon activation:

- **GPCRs:** Activate secondary messengers (cAMP, IP3, DAG) via G proteins
- **Integrins:** Mediate outside-in signaling for cytoskeletal rearrangement
- **Tyrosine Kinase-linked Receptors:** Lead to phosphorylation cascades and granule secretion

These actions lead to:

- Shape change
- Granule secretion (ADP, serotonin, thromboxane)
- Aggregation via fibrinogen bridges
- Clot formation and stabilization

5. Therapeutic Indications

Drugs targeting platelet receptors are essential in preventing and treating thrombotic disorders:

I. **Antiplatelet Therapy in Cardiovascular Diseases**
   - **P2Y12 antagonists:** Clopidogrel, prasugrel, ticagrelor (prevent ADP-mediated aggregation)
   - **GPIIb/IIIa inhibitors:** Abciximab, eptifibatide (block final common pathway of aggregation)
   - **PAR-1 antagonist:** Vorapaxar (thrombin receptor antagonist)
   - **Aspirin:** Inhibits thromboxane A2 synthesis, indirectly affecting TP receptor

II. **Stroke and Transient Ischemic Attack (TIA)**
   - P2Y12 inhibitors and aspirin reduce risk of secondary events

III. **Percutaneous Coronary Interventions (PCI)**
- ❖ Dual antiplatelet therapy (DAPT) involving aspirin and P2Y12 inhibitors

6. Contraindications and Precautions

Antiplatelet therapy targeting platelet receptors should be cautiously administered in:

- ❖ **Active Bleeding:** Absolute contraindication
- ❖ **History of Hemorrhagic Stroke:** Increased risk of intracranial bleeding
- ❖ **Thrombocytopenia:** Risk of bleeding with GPIIb/IIIa inhibitors
- ❖ **Surgery or Trauma:** Risk of perioperative bleeding
- ❖ **Liver Dysfunction:** Affects drug metabolism (e.g., clopidogrel)
- ❖ **Drug Interactions:** Concurrent anticoagulant use increases bleeding risk

7. Summary

Platelet receptors play a central role in hemostasis and pathological thrombosis. Targeting these receptors with pharmacological agents has revolutionized the management of cardiovascular diseases. However, careful assessment of bleeding risk and patient-specific factors is essential for optimizing outcomes.

References

1. Gachet, C. (2006). Regulation of platelet functions by P2 receptors. *Annual Review of Pharmacology and Toxicology*, 46, 277–300.
2. Jackson, S. P. (2007). The growing complexity of platelet aggregation. *Blood*, 109(12), 5087–5095.
3. Clemetson, K. J. (2012). Platelets and primary haemostasis. *Thrombosis Research*, 129(3), 220–224.
4. Bhatt, D. L., & Topol, E. J. (2003). Scientific and clinical aspects of antiplatelet therapy. *Circulation*, 108(25), 2582–2591.
5. Ruggeri, Z. M. (2002). Platelets in atherothrombosis. *Nature Medicine*, 8(11), 1227–1234.

CHAPTER 50

PROLACTIN RECEPTORS: STRUCTURE, SIGNALING MECHANISMS, AND CLINICAL APPLICATIONS

1. Introduction

Prolactin (PRL) is a peptide hormone predominantly known for its role in lactation, but it also regulates a wide array of physiological processes such as immune response, metabolism, and reproduction. These actions are mediated through prolactin receptors (PRLRs), which are widely expressed in various tissues. Understanding PRLR signaling is vital for addressing endocrine, reproductive, and oncologic disorders.

2. Definition

Prolactin receptors are transmembrane proteins belonging to the class I cytokine receptor family. Upon prolactin binding, they initiate intracellular signaling cascades primarily through the Janus kinase-signal transducer and activator of transcription (JAK-STAT) pathway, modulating gene expression related to cell growth, survival, and differentiation.

3. Classification

PRLRs do not have multiple subtypes like some GPCRs, but they exist in different isoforms due to alternative splicing:

A. **Long Form (LF-PRLR):** Fully functional with robust signal transduction capability via JAK2-STAT5.
B. **Intermediate Form (IF-PRLR):** Variably active, with partial signaling competence.
C. **Short Form (SF-PRLR):** May modulate or inhibit signaling; important in tissue-specific regulation.

The receptor isoforms are species-specific and exhibit tissue-specific expression.

4. Pharmacological Actions

Upon prolactin binding, PRLRs dimerize and activate associated JAK2 kinases, which in turn phosphorylate tyrosine residues on the receptor. These phosphorylated sites recruit and activate STAT5, STAT3, or STAT1 transcription factors, leading to nuclear translocation and gene transcription.

Downstream effects include:

- Mammary gland development and lactogenesis
- Immune modulation (e.g., lymphocyte proliferation)
- Neuroprotective functions
- Regulation of reproductive behaviors and metabolism

Pharmacological Modulation:

- **Agonists:** No direct PRLR agonists in clinical use; prolactin is the natural ligand.
- **Antagonists:** Not clinically available yet but under research for treating prolactinomas and PRLR-positive cancers.
- **Dopamine Agonists (e.g., cabergoline, bromocriptine):** Indirectly reduce prolactin levels by inhibiting secretion from the pituitary.

5. Therapeutic Indications

Targeting the PRL-PRLR axis or modulating prolactin secretion is relevant in the management of several conditions:

I. **Hyperprolactinemia**: Treated with dopamine agonists
II. **Prolactinomas**: Pituitary adenomas secreting prolactin; managed pharmacologically and surgically
III. **Infertility and Amenorrhea**: Related to prolactin excess
IV. **Lactation Induction**: Research ongoing into controlled stimulation of PRLR
V. **Breast and Prostate Cancers**: PRLR overexpression associated with poor prognosis; targeted therapies are being explored

6. Contraindications and Precautions

There are no direct PRLR-targeting drugs in routine clinical use yet. However, conditions related to prolactin modulation via dopamine agonists must be considered:

- **Cardiovascular Disease**: Dopamine agonists may exacerbate valvular heart disease
- **Psychiatric Disorders**: Cabergoline and bromocriptine can worsen impulse control disorders or cause hallucinations
- **Pregnancy**: Dopamine agonists usually discontinued during pregnancy unless tumor control is required
- **Pituitary Apoplexy Risk**: In macroprolactinomas, rapid tumor shrinkage may precipitate pituitary apoplexy

7. Summary

Prolactin receptors play an essential role in diverse physiological functions, especially in the reproductive and immune systems. While direct receptor-targeting drugs are still in the experimental stage, modulation of prolactin secretion provides significant therapeutic benefit. Future developments in PRLR antagonism may offer novel treatments for hormone-dependent cancers and autoimmune conditions.

References

1. Bole-Feysot, C., Goffin, V., Edery, M., Binart, N., & Kelly, P. A. (1998). Prolactin (PRL) and its receptor: Actions, signal transduction pathways and phenotypes observed in PRL receptor knockout mice. *Endocrine Reviews*, 19(3), 225–268.
2. Goffin, V., Binart, N., Touraine, P., & Kelly, P. A. (2002). Prolactin: The new biology of an old hormone. *Annual Review of Physiology*, 64, 47–67.
3. Bernard, V., Young, J., Binart, N. (2015). Prolactin—a pleiotropic hormone. *Annals of Endocrinology*, 76(3), 142–147.
4. Larkin, S., & Harvey, S. (2000). Role of prolactin in the immune system. *Journal of Endocrinology*, 168(3), 363–379.
5. Goffin, V., Touraine, P., & Kelly, P. A. (2006). Prolactin receptor antagonists: A new tool in prolactin research. *Trends in Endocrinology & Metabolism*, 17(3), 106–111.

CHAPTER 51

PROSTANOID RECEPTORS

1. Introduction

Prostanoid receptors are a subset of G protein-coupled receptors (GPCRs) that mediate the effects of prostanoids—lipid compounds derived from arachidonic acid via the cyclooxygenase (COX) pathway. These receptors are critical in regulating inflammation, vascular tone, platelet aggregation, and other physiological and pathological processes.

2. Definition

Prostanoid receptors are membrane-bound GPCRs that bind to specific prostanoids such as prostaglandins (PGD_2, PGE_2, $PGF_{2}\alpha$), prostacyclin (PGI_2), and thromboxane A_2 (TXA_2). Upon activation, they initiate intracellular signaling cascades that mediate a variety of biological responses.

3. Classification

Prostanoid receptors are classified into five main types based on their primary ligand affinity:

Receptor	Primary Ligand	Signaling Pathway
DP (DP1, DP2)	PGD_2	DP1 → ↑cAMP (Gs); DP2 (CRTH2) → ↓cAMP, ↑Ca^{2+} (Gi)
EP (EP1, EP2, EP3, EP4)	PGE_2	EP1 → ↑Ca^{2+} (Gq); EP2/EP4 → ↑cAMP (Gs); EP3 → ↓cAMP (Gi)
FP	$PGF_{2}\alpha$	↑Ca^{2+} (Gq)
IP	PGI_2 (prostacyclin)	↑cAMP (Gs)
TP	TXA_2	↑Ca^{2+}, ↓cAMP (Gq, G12/13)

Each receptor subtype shows tissue-specific expression and pharmacological properties, resulting in diverse physiological roles.

4. Pharmacological Actions

DP Receptors:

- ❖ **DP1:** Vasodilation, inhibition of platelet aggregation, sleep regulation.
- ❖ **DP2 (CRTH2):** Chemotaxis of eosinophils and Th2 lymphocytes; involved in allergic inflammation.

EP Receptors:

- ❖ **EP1:** Smooth muscle contraction; involved in pain and fever.
- ❖ **EP2/EP4:** Vasodilation, inhibition of gastric acid secretion, bone formation.
- ❖ **EP3:** Uterine contraction, inhibition of lipolysis, reduction of gastric emptying.

FP Receptors: Uterine smooth muscle contraction, regulation of intraocular pressure.

IP Receptors: Vasodilation, inhibition of platelet aggregation, anti-proliferative effects on vascular smooth muscle.

TP Receptors: Platelet aggregation, bronchoconstriction, vasoconstriction.

5. Therapeutic Indications

Prostanoid receptor-targeting drugs are used in:

1. **Obstetrics and Gynecology**
   - ❖ **Dinoprostone (PGE_2):** Cervical ripening, labor induction (EP receptors).
   - ❖ **Carboprost ($PGF_2\alpha$):** Postpartum hemorrhage (FP receptors).
   - ❖ **Misoprostol (PGE_1 analogue):** Abortifacient and gastric protection.
2. **Cardiovascular Diseases**
   - ❖ **Epoprostenol, iloprost (PGI_2 analogues):** Pulmonary arterial hypertension (IP receptor agonists).
   - ❖ **Aspirin:** Irreversible COX inhibition reduces TXA_2, decreasing platelet aggregation via TP receptor antagonism.
3. **Glaucoma**
   - ❖ **Latanoprost, bimatoprost:** Reduce intraocular pressure (FP receptor agonists).

4. Inflammation and Allergy

- ❖ **DP2 receptor antagonists:** Under investigation for asthma and allergic rhinitis.

6. Contraindications and Precautions

Contraindications may include:

- ❖ **Prostaglandin analogues in pregnancy:** Except for labor induction/abortion (can cause miscarriage).
- ❖ **Asthma:** Some prostanoids may induce bronchospasm (e.g., FP or TP agonists).
- ❖ **Bleeding disorders:** Agents that inhibit TXA_2 (e.g., aspirin) increase bleeding risk.
- ❖ **Hypotension or cardiovascular disease:** Vasodilatory prostanoids like epoprostenol may exacerbate symptoms.

Drug Interactions:

- ❖ NSAIDs and COX inhibitors may blunt the effects of prostanoid analogues.
- ❖ Concurrent anticoagulant therapy increases bleeding risk when using TP receptor antagonists.

7. Summary

Prostanoid receptors represent a diverse and functionally significant family of GPCRs involved in multiple physiological systems. Their pharmacological targeting has yielded critical therapies for cardiovascular, gynecological, ocular, and inflammatory diseases. Ongoing research is expanding the therapeutic landscape through receptor subtype-specific modulators.

References

1. Narumiya, S., Sugimoto, Y., &Ushikubi, F. (1999). Prostanoid receptors: structures, properties, and functions. *Physiological Reviews*, 79(4), 1193–1226.
2. Woodward, D. F., Jones, R. L., &Narumiya, S. (2011). International Union of Basic and Clinical Pharmacology. LXXXIII: Classification of

prostanoid receptors, updating 15 years of progress. *Pharmacological Reviews*, 63(3), 471–538.

3. Coleman, R. A., Smith, W. L., &Narumiya, S. (1994). International Union of Pharmacology classification of prostanoid receptors: properties, distribution, and structure of the receptors and their subtypes. *Pharmacological Reviews*, 46(2), 205–229.
4. Rao, P., & Knaus, E. E. (2008). Evolution of nonsteroidal anti-inflammatory drugs (NSAIDs): cyclooxygenase (COX) inhibition and beyond. *Journal of Pharmacy & Pharmaceutical Sciences*, 11(2), 81–110.
5. Bousquet, J., et al. (2010). CRTH2 antagonists in allergic diseases. *Allergy*, 65(6), 666–668.

CHAPTER 52

QRFP RECEPTORS

1. Introduction

QRFP (also known as 26RFa or pyroglutamylatedRFamide peptide) receptors belong to the RFamide family of neuropeptide receptors. These receptors are involved in the regulation of energy homeostasis, food intake, cardiovascular functions, and reproductive hormone release. QRFP binds primarily to GPR103 (also referred to as QRFPR), a G protein-coupled receptor (GPCR) predominantly expressed in the brain and peripheral tissues.

2. Definition

QRFP receptors are G protein-coupled receptors that bind QRFP neuropeptides (notably 26RFa and 43RFa). These neuropeptides are characterized by a common C-terminal Arg–Phe–NH_2 motif. QRFP receptors play roles in appetite regulation, energy balance, and neuroendocrine signaling.

3. Classification

QRFP receptors belong to the class A (rhodopsin-like) GPCRs and are part of the RFamide receptor family, which includes:

A. **NPFFR1 (GPR147)**
B. **NPFFR2 (GPR74)**
C. **GPR103 (QRFPR) – QRFP-specific receptor**

The main endogenous ligands include:

- **26RFa** (a 26-amino acid peptide)
- **43RFa** (an extended form of 26RFa)

4. Pharmacological Actions

Upon binding of QRFP to GPR103:

Signal transduction is primarily mediated through Gq/11 and Gi/o proteins, leading to:

- o Increased intracellular calcium levels
- o Inhibition of cAMP accumulation
- o Activation of MAPK/ERK pathways

Physiological roles include:

- ❖ **Appetite stimulation** and increased food intake
- ❖ **Regulation of body weight** and fat deposition
- ❖ **Modulation of blood pressure and heart rate**
- ❖ **Stimulation of gonadotropin-releasing hormone (GnRH) secretion**
- ❖ **Interaction with orexigenic and anorexigenic neurocircuits**

Experimental models have shown that intracerebroventricular administration of QRFP peptides increases food consumption and alters neuroendocrine hormone levels.

5. Therapeutic Indications

While QRFP-targeted therapies are still under investigation, potential indications include:

- ❖ **Obesity and metabolic disorders** – due to their orexigenic (appetite-promoting) effect
- ❖ **Reproductive hormone dysregulation** – QRFP has a role in the hypothalamic-pituitary-gonadal axis
- ❖ **Hypertension and cardiovascular modulation** – via central nervous system pathways

6. Contraindications and Precautions

Since no QRFP-targeting drugs are currently approved, contraindications **are theoretical or based on biological plausibility:**

- ❖ **Obesity or metabolic syndrome**: Agonists could exacerbate energy imbalance

- ❖ **Hormone-sensitive conditions**: Caution in diseases affected by altered GnRH levels
- ❖ **Hypertension or cardiovascular disease**: Central QRFP activity might influence blood pressure regulation

Further clinical trials are required to establish safety and efficacy in human populations.

7. Summary

QRFP receptors, primarily represented by GPR103, are novel neuromodulatory receptors involved in metabolic, reproductive, and cardiovascular regulation. While pharmacological modulation is not yet part of standard therapy, their emerging role in energy balance and endocrine signaling highlights them as promising targets for future drug development.

References

1. Chartrel, N., et al. (2003). Identification of 26RFa, a hypothalamic neuropeptide of the RFamide peptide family with orexigenic activity. *Proceedings of the National Academy of Sciences*, 100(24), 15247–15252.
2. Fukusumi, S., et al. (2003). A new peptidic ligand and its receptor regulating adrenal function in rats. *The Journal of Biological Chemistry*, 278(46), 46387–46395.
3. Leprince, J., et al. (2009). 26RFa and its role in the control of energy homeostasis. *Peptides*, 30(11), 1894–1901.
4. Takayasu, S., et al. (2006). Distribution of the mRNA for a G-protein-coupled receptor for the RFamide-related peptide, 26RFa, in the rat brain. *Brain Research*, 1070(1), 45–52.
5. Mounien, L., et al. (2010). The hypothalamic neuropeptide 26RFa (QRFP) and its role in the regulation of food intake. *Frontiers in Endocrinology*, 1, 14.

CHAPTER 53

SOMATOSTATIN RECEPTORS

1. Introduction

Somatostatin, a neuropeptide hormone, plays a vital role in the inhibition of endocrine and exocrine secretions, neurotransmission, and cellular proliferation. The biological actions of somatostatin are mediated by a family of G protein-coupled receptors (GPCRs) known as somatostatin receptors (SSTRs). These receptors are widely expressed in the central nervous system, gastrointestinal tract, pancreas, and several endocrine and non-endocrine tissues.

2. Definition

Somatostatin receptors (SSTRs) are a group of five high-affinity GPCRs (SSTR1 to SSTR5) that mediate the inhibitory effects of somatostatin on hormone secretion, cell proliferation, and neurotransmission. They exert their actions via inhibition of adenylyl cyclase, modulation of calcium and potassium channels, and activation of phosphotyrosine phosphatases.

3. Classification

Somatostatin receptors are classified into **five subtypes** based on gene structure, binding affinity, and pharmacological properties:

Receptor Subtype	Tissue Expression	Functions
SSTR1	Brain, gastrointestinal tract	Inhibits growth hormone release, synaptic transmission
SSTR2	Widely expressed; especially pancreas, pituitary	Strongly inhibits GH and insulin secretion

SSTR3	Brain, kidney, pancreatic islets	Induces apoptosis
SSTR4	Brain, lung	Pain modulation, anti-inflammatory roles
SSTR5	Pancreas, pituitary	Inhibits insulin and GH secretion

4. Pharmacological Actions

SSTRs mediate somatostatin's inhibitory effects through:

- **Inhibition of adenylyl cyclase** → ↓ cAMP
- **Modulation of ion channels** → ↓ calcium influx, ↑ potassium efflux
- **Inhibition of hormone secretion**: GH, insulin, glucagon, TSH, gastrin
- **Anti-proliferative effects**: via activation of phosphotyrosine phosphatases and p53
- **Apoptosis induction** (notably via SSTR3)
- **Modulation of neurotransmitter release** in the CNS

Synthetic analogs like octreotide and lanreotide act preferentially on SSTR2 and SSTR5.

5. Therapeutic Indications

Somatostatin receptor agonists (e.g., octreotide, lanreotide, pasireotide) are clinically used for:

Endocrine Disorders

- **Acromegaly**: suppression of GH in pituitary adenomas (SSTR2, SSTR5)
- **Cushing's disease**: suppression of ACTH (pasireotide → SSTR1,2,3,5)

Neuroendocrine Tumors

- Carcinoid syndrome, gastrinoma, VIPoma, glucagonoma
- Symptom control and tumor growth inhibition

Gastrointestinal Bleeding

- ❖ Esophageal variceal hemorrhage (vasoconstriction and reduced portal pressure)

Radiolabeled Diagnostic Imaging and Therapy

- ❖ SSTR-targeted imaging (e.g., ^68Ga-DOTATATE PET) and radionuclide therapy (e.g., ^177Lu-DOTATATE)

6. Contraindications and Precautions

Use of somatostatin analogs is contraindicated or requires caution in:

- **Known hypersensitivity** to somatostatin or analogs
- **Gallbladder disease**: Risk of biliary sludge and cholelithiasis
- **Diabetes mellitus**: Can worsen glucose control (due to insulin and glucagon inhibition)
- **Bradycardia or conduction abnormalities**
- **Renal and hepatic impairment**: Requires dose adjustment

7. Summary

Somatostatin receptors are crucial regulators of hormone secretion, cell growth, and neurotransmission. Pharmacological modulation of these receptors has transformed the management of acromegaly, neuroendocrine tumors, and other endocrine disorders. Ongoing research continues to explore the therapeutic potential of targeting individual SSTR subtypes.

References

1. Patel, Y. C. (1999). Somatostatin and its receptor family. *Frontiers in Neuroendocrinology*, 20(3), 157–198. https://doi.org/10.1006/frne.1999.0183
2. Schally, A. V., & Nagy, A. (2004). Cancer chemotherapy based on targeting of cytotoxic peptide conjugates to their receptors. *European Journal of Endocrinology*, 151(1), T11–T17.
3. Hofland, L. J., & Lamberts, S. W. (2003). The pathophysiological consequences of somatostatin receptor internalization and resistance. *Endocrine Reviews*, 24(1), 28–47.
4. Reubi, J. C. (2003). Peptide receptors as molecular targets for cancer diagnosis and therapy. *Endocrine Reviews*, 24(4), 389–427.
5. Cives, M., &Strosberg, J. R. (2018). Gastroenteropancreatic neuroendocrine tumors. *CA: A Cancer Journal for Clinicians*, 68(6), 471–487. https://doi.org/10.3322/caac.21494

CHAPTER 54

SUCCINATE RECEPTORS

1. Definition

Succinate receptors, primarily represented by SUCNR1 (also known as GPR91), are G protein-coupled receptors (GPCRs) activated by succinate, a citric acid cycle (TCA cycle) intermediate. SUCNR1 functions as a metabolic sensor that links cellular energy status with physiological responses such as inflammation, blood pressure regulation, and retinal angiogenesis.

2. Classification

- **Family**: G protein-coupled receptors (Class A, rhodopsin-like)
- **Receptor**: SUCNR1 (formerly GPR91)
- **Endogenous Ligand**: Succinate (a dicarboxylic acid metabolite)
- **Signaling Pathways**: Primarily through **Gq** and **Gi/o** proteins

3. Pharmacological Actions

Upon succinate binding, SUCNR1 activation leads to:

- **Intracellular calcium mobilization** via **Gq pathway**
- **Inhibition of adenylate cyclase** via **Gi/o**, leading to ↓ cAMP
- **MAPK and ERK pathway activation**
- **Reactive oxygen species (ROS) generation**

Physiological and pathophysiological actions:

- **Renin release and blood pressure regulation** (kidneys)
- **Modulation of immune response** (dendritic cells, macrophages)
- **Retinal angiogenesis** (important in diabetic retinopathy)
- **Fibrosis and inflammation** in liver and adipose tissue
- **Stimulation of erythropoietin** production during hypoxia

4. Therapeutic Indications

While no SUCNR1-targeting drugs are clinically approved yet, potential therapeutic areas include:

- **Hypertension and Renal Disorders**
  - Due to succinate-mediated renin release and renal signaling
- **Metabolic Syndrome and Obesity**
  - Succinate levels rise with mitochondrial dysfunction; targeting SUCNR1 may mitigate inflammation
- **Diabetic Retinopathy**
  - Excessive succinate in the retina stimulates abnormal angiogenesis
- **Liver Fibrosis / NAFLD**
  - SUCNR1 contributes to hepatic inflammation and fibrogenesis
- **Autoimmune and Inflammatory Diseases**
  - Modulating immune cell activation via SUCNR1

5. Contraindications and Precautions

Since no drugs directly targeting SUCNR1 are approved yet, contraindications are theoretical:

- **Systemic Immunosuppression**: Blocking SUCNR1 may suppress immune surveillance
- **Hypotension Risk**: Inhibiting SUCNR1 may impair renin-angiotensin system function
- **Ocular Effects**: Inhibition could affect physiological angiogenesis in retinal tissue

Caution is advised in preclinical research due to tissue-specific and context-dependent roles of SUCNR1.

6. Summary

Succinate receptors, especially SUCNR1, function as metabolic sensors that integrate mitochondrial status with systemic physiological responses. Their role in inflammation, angiogenesis, and metabolism makes them promising targets for a range of chronic diseases. Further research is ongoing to develop selective SUCNR1 modulators for clinical use.

Classification

Feature	Details
Receptor Name	SUCNR1 (Succinate Receptor 1)
Other Name	GPR91
Receptor Type	G protein-coupled receptor (Class A)
Endogenous Ligand	Succinate
Signaling Pathways	Gi/o, Gq, MAPK

3. Pharmacological Actions

Upon succinate binding, SUCNR1 activates intracellular signaling cascades involving:

- ❖ **Gi/o protein coupling**: Inhibits adenylate cyclase → ↓ cAMP levels.
- ❖ **Gq coupling**: Activates phospholipase C (PLC) → ↑ IP_3 and DAG → ↑ intracellular calcium.
- ❖ **MAPK/ERK pathways:** Promotes cell proliferation, angiogenesis, and inflammatory responses.

Functional Outcomes:

- ❖ Promotes **renin release** in juxtaglomerular cells (blood pressure regulation).
- ❖ Stimulates **angiogenesis** in hypoxic tissues, especially the retina.
- ❖ Enhances **pro-inflammatory cytokine** production in macrophages and dendritic cells.
- ❖ Modulates **fibrogenic activity** in the liver and adipose tissue.
- ❖ Acts as a **metabolic sensor** in conditions like hypoxia, ischemia, and oxidative stress.

4. Therapeutic Indications (Potential/Investigational)

Though there are currently no approved SUCNR1-targeting drugs, several potential applications are under investigation:

a. Diabetic Retinopathy: SUCNR1 mediates retinal neovascularization by sensing local succinate accumulation.

b. Hypertension: Via renin-angiotensin system activation; potential target to modulate BP.

c. Metabolic Syndrome and Obesity: Succinate acts as a danger signal; SUCNR1 contributes to adipose tissue inflammation and insulin resistance.

d. Liver Fibrosis / Non-Alcoholic Fatty Liver Disease (NAFLD): Involved in hepatic stellate cell activation and fibrosis progression.

e. Rheumatoid Arthritis: Activation of SUCNR1 on immune cells augments inflammation in joints.

5. Contraindications and Precautions

As SUCNR1 modulators are still in the experimental stage, the following are **theoretical risks** associated with modulation:

- ❖ **Risk of Immunosuppression**: Inhibiting SUCNR1 may suppress beneficial immune responses.
- ❖ **Renal Hypotension**: Antagonism may reduce renin release and impair blood pressure homeostasis.
- ❖ **Retinal Health**: Inhibition may affect physiological angiogenesis, particularly in ischemic retinal diseases.
- ❖ **Metabolic Disturbances**: Long-term SUCNR1 antagonism may affect insulin-glucose regulation.

Precaution: Drug targeting SUCNR1 must be tissue-specific and condition-specific due to its **pleiotropic roles** in various systems.

6. Summary

Succinate receptor SUCNR1 is a pivotal link between metabolic disturbances and immune-inflammatory responses. It holds promise as a therapeutic target in metabolic, cardiovascular, hepatic, and ocular diseases. Ongoing research aims to develop selective agonists or antagonists for clinical intervention in diseases characterized by oxidative stress and mitochondrial dysfunction.

References

1. He, W., et al. (2004). Citric acid cycle intermediates as ligands for orphan G-protein–coupled receptors. *Nature*, 429(6988), 188–193. https://doi.org/10.1038/nature02488

2. Toma, I., & Sipos, A. (2011). GPR91: a new player in the pathogenesis of diabetic nephropathy. *American Journal of Physiology-Renal Physiology*, 300(2), F375–F381.
3. Littlewood-Evans, A., et al. (2016). GPR91 senses extracellular succinate released from inflammatory macrophages and exacerbates rheumatoid arthritis. *The Journal of Experimental Medicine*, 213(9), 1655–1662.
4. Mills, E. L., et al. (2016). Succinate dehydrogenase supports metabolic repurposing of mitochondria to drive inflammatory macrophages. *Cell*, 167(2), 457–470.e13.
5. Aguiar, C. J., et al. (2010). Succinate causes cardiomyocyte hypertrophy through GPR91 activation. *Cell Communication and Signaling*, 8, 23.
6. He, W., et al. (2004). Citric acid cycle intermediates as ligands for orphan G-protein–coupled receptors. *Nature*, 429(6988), 188–193. https://doi.org/10.1038/nature02488
7. Toma, I., & Sipos, A. (2011). GPR91: a new player in the pathogenesis of diabetic nephropathy. *American Journal of Physiology-Renal Physiology*, 300(2), F375–F381.
8. Robben, J. H., et al. (2009). Hypotension and reduced aldosterone levels in mice lacking GPR91. *Kidney International*, 75(9), 898–906.
9. Littlewood-Evans, A., et al. (2016). GPR91 senses extracellular succinate released from inflammatory macrophages and exacerbates rheumatoid arthritis. *The Journal of Experimental Medicine*, 213(9), 1655–1662.
10. Aguiar, C. J., et al. (2010). Succinate causes cardiomyocyte hypertrophy through GPR91 activation. *Cell Communication and Signaling*, 8, 23.

CHAPTER 55

TACHYKININ RECEPTORS

1. Definition

Tachykinin receptors are a subgroup of G protein-coupled receptors (GPCRs) that mediate the physiological and pathophysiological actions of tachykinins, a family of neuropeptides. The most well-known tachykinins include substance P, neurokinin A, and neurokinin B. These peptides are involved in nociception, inflammation, smooth muscle contraction, and neuroimmune communication.

2. Classification

Tachykinin receptors are classified into three main subtypes based on their endogenous ligands and sequence homology:

Receptor	Preferred Ligand	Gene Symbol	Distribution
NK1 (Neurokinin 1)	Substance P	TACR1	CNS, GIT, cardiovascular and immune system
NK2 (Neurokinin 2)	Neurokinin A	TACR2	GIT, bladder, uterus, spinal cord
NK3 (Neurokinin 3)	Neurokinin B	TACR3	Hypothalamus, basal ganglia, peripheral nerves

All three are **Class A (rhodopsin-like) GPCRs** that couple primarily to **Gq/11 proteins**, leading to activation of phospholipase C, calcium mobilization, and downstream protein kinase signaling.

3. Pharmacological Actions

a. Signal Transduction

- **Gq/11 pathway activation** → PLC-β → IP_3 + DAG → ↑ intracellular Ca^{2+} → PKC activation
- Modulation of other pathways: MAPK/ERK, PI3K/Akt in specific tissues

b. Physiological Effects

A. **NK1 Receptors**:
  - Mediates pain perception, emesis, inflammation, and vasodilation
  - Promotes neurogenic inflammation by activating mast cells and releasing cytokines

B. **NK2 Receptors**:
  - Induce smooth muscle contraction, especially in the gastrointestinal tract and airways
  - Involved in bronchoconstriction and visceral pain

C. **NK3 Receptors**:
  - Involved in central neuroendocrine regulation, thermoregulation, and behavior
  - Important for reproductive hormone release via GnRH modulation

4. Therapeutic Indications

Several NK receptor antagonists have been developed for various clinical conditions, particularly NK1 receptor antagonists:

Table

Indication	**Receptor Targeted**	**Examples of Drugs**
Chemotherapy-induced nausea and vomiting (CINV)	NK1	Aprepitant, Fosaprepitant
Post-operative nausea and vomiting (PONV)	NK1	Rolapitant, Netupitant
Major depressive disorder (MDD)*(experimental)*	NK1	Aprepitant (investigational)
Asthma, COPD *(investigational)*	NK2	Nepadutant, Saredutant

Irritable Bowel Syndrome (IBS)*(investigational)*	NK2	Ibodutant
Hot flashes, menopausal symptoms	NK3	Fezolinetant

5. Contraindications and Precautions

Though generally well tolerated, NK receptor antagonists carry specific cautions:

Condition	**Concern**
Hepatic Impairment	Drugs like aprepitant are hepatically metabolized
Drug Interactions (CYP3A4)	NK1 antagonists inhibit CYP3A4; potential for interactions with warfarin, midazolam, dexamethasone
Pregnancy and Lactation	Safety not well established for NK receptor antagonists
Hypersensitivity	Rare allergic reactions to tachykinin receptor drugs
Depression or psychiatric illness	Some NK1 antagonists were investigated but discontinued due to adverse psychiatric effects

6. Summary

Tachykinin receptors are essential mediators of neuropeptide signaling across a range of physiological and pathophysiological processes. Pharmacological modulation of NK receptors, especially NK1, has led to the development of important antiemetic agents, with ongoing research into roles in inflammation, pain, depression, and hormonal regulation. Continued exploration of NK2 and NK3 receptor modulators may offer novel therapeutic avenues for respiratory, gastrointestinal, and neuroendocrine disorders.

References

1. Quartara, L., & Maggi, C. A. (1998). The tachykinin NK1 receptor. *Part I: Ligands and mechanisms of cellular activation. Neuropeptides*, 32(1), 1–49.
2. Rupniak, N. M., & Kramer, M. S. (1999). Discovery of the antidepressant and anti-emetic efficacy of substance P receptor (NK1) antagonists. *Trends in Pharmacological Sciences*, 20(12), 485–490.

3. Patacchini, R., & Maggi, C. A. (2001). Tachykinin receptor antagonists in clinical trials. *Drug News & Perspectives*, 14(6), 373–380.
4. Doods, H. N., et al. (2007). Therapeutic potential of tachykinin NK2 receptor antagonists in the treatment of functional bowel disorders. *Neurogastroenterology& Motility*, 19(5), 313–319.
5. Fraser, G. L., et al. (2020). Fezolinetant (ESN364), a selective neurokinin-3 receptor antagonist for the treatment of vasomotor symptoms associated with menopause. *The Lancet*, 396(10253), 1203–1214.

CHAPTER 56

THYROTROPIN RECEPTORS (TSH RECEPTORS)

1. Definition

Thyrotropin receptors (TSHR) are specific **G protein-coupled receptors (GPCRs)** located primarily on the surface of thyroid follicular cells. They mediate the actions of **thyroid-stimulating hormone (TSH)**, a pituitary hormone responsible for regulating thyroid gland growth and the synthesis and release of thyroid hormones (T_3 and T_4).

2. Classification

Feature	Details
Receptor Name	Thyrotropin receptor (TSHR)
Receptor Type	G protein-coupled receptor (Class A, rhodopsin-like)
Gene Symbol	**TSHR**
Endogenous Ligand	Thyroid-stimulating hormone (TSH)
Primary Tissue Expression	Thyroid follicular cells, also in adipose and bone
G Protein Coupling	Primarily **Gs**, also **Gq** in some contexts

3. Pharmacological Actions

a. Signal Transduction

- **Gs pathway activation** → ↑ Adenylate cyclase → ↑ cAMP → ↑ PKA → Transcription of thyroid hormone synthesis genes.
- **Gq pathway (minor)** → Activation of phospholipase C (PLC) → ↑ IP_3 and DAG → ↑ intracellular calcium.

b. Physiological Effects

- **Stimulation of iodide uptake** (via NIS transporter)
- **Activation of thyroglobulin iodination** and hormone synthesis
- **Promotion of T_3 and T_4 release**
- **Thyroid cell growth and proliferation** (trophic effect)

4. Indications for Targeting TSHR

Although no direct TSHR agonists or antagonists are widely used clinically, TSH receptor modulation is relevant in several diagnostic and therapeutic contexts:

a. Diagnostic Use

- **Recombinant human TSH (rhTSH)** (e.g., **Thyrogen®**):
  - Used to stimulate thyroid tissue in **thyroid cancer follow-up** or **radioiodine ablation**.

b. Autoimmunity & Therapeutic Targets

- TSHR is the autoantigen in Graves' disease: Stimulating autoantibodies mimic TSH, causing hyperthyroidism.
- Investigational therapies target TSHR-blocking antibodies or small molecule antagonists for autoimmune thyroid diseases.

5. Contraindications and Precautions

a. rhTSH Use (e.g., Thyrogen®)

Condition	Concern
Adrenal insufficiency	May exacerbate metabolic instability
Uncontrolled thyrotoxicosis	Stimulation may worsen hyperthyroid symptoms
Pregnancy/Lactation	Use with caution; thyroid hormone regulation is crucial
Allergy to recombinant proteins	Hypersensitivity reactions possible

b. TSHR-Stimulating Antibodies (Pathological Context)

- **Graves' Disease**: Contraindicates use of TSH or agents that increase TSH.
- **TSHR-blocking antibodies** (rare): Can cause **hypothyroidism** by inhibiting endogenous TSH signaling.

6. Summary

Thyrotropin receptors (TSHR) play a central role in thyroid physiology and are critically involved in both normal endocrine function and thyroid autoimmune diseases such as Graves' disease. While therapeutic manipulation of TSHR is limited to recombinant TSH and experimental agents, its diagnostic and pathophysiological relevance is profound.

References

1. Davies, T. F., & Latif, R. (2002). The TSH receptor and thyroid autoimmunity: insights into receptor structure and function. *Endocrine Reviews*, 23(2), 223–246.
2. Rapoport, B., & McLachlan, S. M. (2014). Thyroid-stimulating hormone receptor autoantibodies. *Endocrinology and Metabolism Clinics*, 43(2), 267–283.
3. Luster, M., et al. (2005). rhTSH in the management of differentiated thyroid cancer: a systematic review. *European Journal of Endocrinology*, 153(6), 651–658.
4. Sanders, J., et al. (2010). A human monoclonal autoantibody to the TSH receptor that blocks stimulating antibodies in Graves' disease. *Thyroid*, 20(10), 1009–1014.

CHAPTER 57

VASOPRESSIN RECEPTORS

1. Definition

Vasopressin receptors are specific **G protein-coupled receptors (GPCRs)** that mediate the physiological and pharmacological actions of **arginine vasopressin (AVP)**, also known as antidiuretic hormone (ADH). These receptors play key roles in regulating water homeostasis, vascular tone, and the release of adrenocorticotropic hormone (ACTH).

2. Classification

There are **three major subtypes** of vasopressin receptors, each encoded by different genes and coupled to distinct intracellular signaling pathways:

Receptor Type	**Gene**	**Location**	**G Protein Coupling**	**Primary Action**
V_1A (V1R)	**AVPR1A**	Vascular smooth muscle, liver, brain	Gq/11	Vasoconstriction, glycogenolysis
V_1B (V3R)	**AVPR1B**	Anterior pituitary, pancreas	Gq/11	ACTH secretion
V_2	**AVPR2**	Renal collecting ducts (principal cells)	Gs	Water reabsorption via aquaporin-2

3. Pharmacological Actions

a. V_1A Receptors

- **Gq protein activation** → ↑ IP_3 and DAG → ↑ intracellular Ca^{2+}
- Causes:
  - **Vasoconstriction** → increased peripheral resistance and blood pressure
  - **Glycogenolysis** in the liver
  - Behavioral and social function modulation in CNS

b. V_1B Receptors

- Found in anterior pituitary corticotrophs
- Stimulates **ACTH release** → ↑ cortisol production from adrenal cortex
- Also involved in insulin and glucagon regulation in pancreas

c. V_2 Receptors

- Gs protein activation → ↑ adenylate cyclase → ↑ cAMP → ↑ PKA
- Induces translocation of aquaporin-2 channels to apical membrane of renal collecting duct → water reabsorption
- Also promotes von Willebrand factor (vWF) and factor VIII release from endothelium

4. Therapeutic Indications

Vasopressin receptor agonists and antagonists are used in several clinical settings:

Agonists

- **Desmopressin (DDAVP)** – selective V_2 agonist:
  - **Central diabetes insipidus**
  - **Nocturnal enuresis**
  - **Mild hemophilia A and von Willebrand disease** (↑ vWF and factor VIII)
- **Vasopressin (AVP)** – mixed V_1/V_2 activity:
  - **Vasodilatory shock** (e.g., septic shock)
  - **Advanced cardiac life support (ACLS)** – as vasopressor

Antagonists

- **Tolvaptan, Conivaptan** – V_2 receptor antagonists (vaptans):
  - **Hyponatremia** (especially SIADH)
  - **Heart failure** with fluid overload

5. Contraindications and Precautions

Drug/Class	Contraindications	Cautions
Desmopressin	-Hyponatremia- Moderate/severe renal impairment	- Fluid intake must be restricted
Vasopressin (AVP)	- Chronic nephritis- Ischemic heart disease	- Risk of coronary vasospasm and arrhythmias
Tolvaptan/Conivaptan	- Hypovolemic hyponatremia- Anuria	- Monitor sodium correction to avoid ODS

ODS = Osmotic Demyelination Syndrome due to rapid correction of sodium

6. Clinical Notes

- **V_1A agonists** are being explored for **vasodilatory shock**, especially when catecholamines fail.
- **V_2 antagonists** are considered aquaretics, meaning they promote free water clearance without electrolyte loss.
- Vasopressin analogshave off-label interest in bleeding disorders due to their procoagulant effects.

7. Summary

Vasopressin receptors are central to the regulation of fluid balance, vascular tone, and stress hormone release. Their pharmacological modulation through selective agonists and antagonists provides essential therapeutic tools in endocrinology, cardiology, and critical care. Understanding receptor subtype-specific actions ensures effective and safe clinical application.

References

1. Verbalis, J. G., Goldsmith, S. R., Greenberg, A., et al. (2013). Diagnosis, evaluation, and treatment of hyponatremia: expert panel recommendations. *The American Journal of Medicine*, 126(10), S1–S42.
2. Holmes, C. L., Landry, D. W., &Granton, J. T. (2004). Science review: Vasopressin and the cardiovascular system. *Critical Care*, 8(6), 427–435.

3. Robertson, G. L. (1985). The regulation of vasopressin function in health and disease. *Recent Progress in Hormone Research*, 41, 473–512.
4. Schrier, R. W. (2006). Vasopressin and aquaporin 2 in clinical disorders of water homeostasis. *Seminars in Nephrology*, 26(3), 290–296.
5. Decaux, G., &Soupart, A. (2008). Treatment of symptomatic hyponatremia. *Best Practice & Research Clinical Endocrinology & Metabolism*, 22(2), 273–285.

CHAPTER 58

OXYTOCIN RECEPTORS

1. Definition

Oxytocin receptors (OXTR) are **G protein-coupled receptors (GPCRs)** that mediate the physiological effects of **oxytocin**, a nonapeptide hormone secreted by the posterior pituitary. These receptors are involved in reproductive physiology, emotional bonding, social behavior, and uterine contractions during labor.

2. Classification

Feature	**Details**
Receptor Name	Oxytocin Receptor (OXTR)
Receptor Type	Class A GPCR
Gene Symbol	**OXTR**
Ligand	Oxytocin
Primary Tissue Expression	Uterus, mammary glands, brain, kidney, heart
G Protein Coupling	**Gq/11**

3. Pharmacological Actions

a. Signal Transduction

- Oxytocin binds to OXTR, activating the **Gq/11 pathway**:
  - ↑ Phospholipase C (PLC) → ↑ IP_3 and DAG
  - ↑ Intracellular calcium → smooth muscle contraction
  - Activation of protein kinase C (PKC)

b. Physiological Effects

- **Uterine contractions** during labor
- **Milk ejection reflex** via contraction of myoepithelial cells in the mammary glands
- Modulation of **social behavior**, stress responses, and pair bonding (central actions in the brain)

4. Therapeutic Indications

Oxytocin Agonists (e.g., Oxytocin injection)

- Induction or augmentation of labor
- Management of postpartumhemorrhage (PPH)
- Promotion of milk let-down (less common clinical use today)

Oxytocin Receptor Antagonists

- **Atosiban** (not widely available in pall countries): Used for **tocolysis** (prevention of preterm labor) in Europe and other regions

5. Contraindications and Precautions

Clinical Use	Contraindications
Oxytocin administration	- Cephalopelvic disproportion- Fetal distress- Malpresentation- Previous uterine surgery (e.g., C-section)- Hypertonic uterus
Atosiban (antagonist)	- Intrauterine fetal demise- Severe preeclampsia- Antepartum hemorrhage requiring delivery

Precautions

- **Risk of uterine hyperstimulation** → fetal hypoxia
- **Water intoxication** at high doses due to oxytocin's antidiuretic effect (similar to vasopressin)
- Monitor fetal heart rate and uterine contractions during oxytocin use

6. Summary

Oxytocin receptors play a pivotal role in reproductive physiology and social neurobiology. Pharmacological modulation of OXTR has critical obstetric applications, especially in labor induction and prevention of postpartum hemorrhage. Clinical use requires careful monitoring to prevent complications such as uterine rupture or fetal distress.

References

1. Gimpl, G., & Fahrenholz, F. (2001). The oxytocin receptor system: structure, function, and regulation. *Physiological Reviews*, 81(2), 629–683.
2. Arrowsmith, S., & Wray, S. (2014). Oxytocin: Its mechanism of action and receptor signalling in the myometrium. *Journal of Neuroendocrinology*, 26(6), 356–369.
3. Moos, W. H., et al. (2017). The therapeutic potential of oxytocin in human health: A review. *Brain Research*, 1654, 12–24.
4. European Medicines Agency. (2015). Assessment report for Atosiban.
5. WHO Model List of Essential Medicines. (2023). Oxytocin.

INDEX